The Cure is in the Cause
Nature's Wisdom and Life Itself

A Guide To:

Health
Happiness
Harmony
Love
Success
Liberty
and
Truth

By
Dr. Ruza Bogdanovich, ND

"Come forth into the light of things, let Nature be your teacher."
William Wordsworth

**The Cure is in the Cause - Nature's Wisdom and Life Itself
By Dr. Ruza Bogdanovich, N.D.**

DISCLAIMER:
This book is sold for educational purposes only. Neither the author nor the publisher will be held accountable for the use or misuse of the information contained in this book. This book is not intended as medical advice because the author and publisher of this work do not recommend the use of prescription drugs or processed foods to alleviate health challenges. Because there is always some risk involved, the author, publisher, and/or distributors of this book are not responsible for any adverse detoxification effects or consequences resulting from the use of any suggestions, recommendations or procedures described hereafter.

ISBN #: 0-9704403-0-8
LC Control Number: 00 092672
First Edition: 2001
Cover Art: Jesse Bogdanovich
Jacket Design: Randy D Johnson, Project X Creative, Reno, NV
Authors photograph © by Jay Aldrich

Copyright © 2001 Ruza V. Bogdanovich
Published by Spirit Spring Foundation, Inc.
Box 53
Genoa, Nevada, U.S.A. 89411
www.thecureisinthecause.org
www.thecureisinthecause.com
drruza@hotmail.com
www.spirit-springs.org

Spirit Spring Foundation Incorporated is a non-profit corporation organized exclusively to develop public awareness and understanding of natural healing processes.

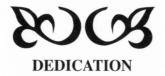

DEDICATION

To the fondest memory of my beloved father and mother who taught me to always search for truth. To my sons, Jesse and Sean, who are the cause of my awakening and a change of career to Naturopathy. To my greatest teacher of all, Nature and awareness of her eternal truth, and to my family, Michael Bogdanovich, my brothers and sisters.

With gratitude to every author, my teachers, the children, especially Luka, all creatures great and small, and microbes, too. I love you all unconditionally.

May you always stay on Nature's path.

Ruza Bogdanovich

"If any man can convince me or bring home to me that I do not think or act o' right, gladly will I change; for I search after the truth by which man never yet was harmed, but he is harmed who abideth on still in his deception and ignorance."

Marcus Aurelius Antonius

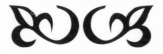

FOREWORD
By Denise S. LaBee

When I first agreed to undertake the editing of this book, I was admittedly skeptical. Being (I thought) well-read, well-informed, capable of differentiating between "real" medicine and hoo-doo quackery, I approached this project with tongue firmly placed in cheek.

Yes, I spent the last twenty years growing herbs, casually studying their uses and touting the benefits of some natural herbal remedies over the synthetics pushed by mainstream medics, but Naturopathy, Iridology, Nature's law of Cause and Effect and raw food diet? Strange creatures indeed.

At first I disagreed with every radical thought and unfamiliar concept, arguing with the words on the computer screen as I typed. As the facts were laid out before me, I began to see the truth in them. The discovery of one truth lead quickly to another. Then came "the moment." Suddenly I found myself agreeing with what was being said - totally, completely, one hundred percent. It was shocking and it was the beginning of an eye-opening, often spiritual journey for me. Because I agreed so readily with one point, I thought, why be so quick to dismiss the others? The truth became self-evident.

What I learned once I opened my mind jolted me into a new reality - real truth. I believe human kind is in deep trouble. We have gotten far out of touch with Nature. Look around you and take heed of Nature's warnings.

All four of my grandparents lived well into their nineties, however my parents both died at relatively young ages, riddled with disease: metastasized cancer, thyroid, diabetes and heart condition. Yet the medical establishment is saying we're living longer now. What will happen to my generation, and the next? What will happen to our Earth? What will our future be like?

What can I do to turn things around. The answers are found in *Nature's Wisdom and Life Itself - The Cure is in the Cause.*

Dr. Ruza Bogdanovich has certainly done her homework. Within the pages of this book are clearly demonstrated the simple, powerful truths of *Nature's Wisdom*, presented in a way that gently and gradually introduces unfamiliar concepts without overwhelming the reader with a cascade of new information.

Built on the solid foundations of such internationally-known Natural Health advocates such as Dr. Bernard Jensen, Dr. John H. Tilden, Dr. Thomas Sydenham, Dr. Robert Bell, Dr. Harvey Kellog, Dr. Richard Lambe, Dr. William Howard Hay, Dr. Alexis Carrel, Dr. Richard Moskowitz, Dr. Robert Mendelsohn, Dr. Alan S. Levin, Dr. Henry Heimlich, Dr. Richard Schulze, Dr. Richard Anderson, Ross Horne, author of many true health books with his latest best seller *Health and Survival in the Twenty-first Century*, the author of *The Sunfood Diet Success System*, David Wolfe, and many other true teachers.

The Cure is in the Cause is an eye-opening, and often spiritual journey for anyone interested in a Natural alternative to prescription medicine and modern life.

In addition to providing a fascinating overview of the various aspects of Nature, health, Natural and Alternative Therapies, this book will take you on an exploration with an appealing simplicity of the wonderful benefits awaiting us all when we achieve our goal of good health: happiness, harmony, love, success, and liberty. This is not a quick fix. This is a change in attitude, a change in lifestyle, and a new commitment to a whole new you.

Dr. Bogdanovich is asking us all, again and again to listen deep and hear a beat of Nature's drum that is our birthright and in all of our best interests. There is hope. Nature's path is the way. Please join me.

A santé.

**Denise S. LaBee, January
2001**

TABLE OF CONTENTS

CHAPTER THREE

CHAPTER EIGHT

CHAPTER NINE

ILLUSTRATIONS

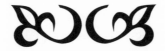

ACKNOWLEDGEMENTS

I wish to acknowledge the immeasurable contribution others have made in my life by sharing their enlightenment with me through their writings, teachings and friendships.

No one writes books alone. Some of the ideas herein are combined from others long forgotten. Some are from a new generation of geniuses like those mentioned throughout this book, and thousands of others whom I have no room to mention. Over time, I've forgotten many in the specifics of who said what, or when I've read about them. *Absence of proof is not proof of absence.* No matter, they touched me deeply. I especially want to thank those unnamed intellects for their persistence and for how they eventually got their point across. I will always be grateful.

The sunlight looks a little different on this wall than it does on that wall and lot different on this other one, but it still one light. One truth.

My work is my passion and a sincere desire to help from the bottom of my heart. I hope that you may only benefit from this knowledge and see the truth in the light of the day so you may confidently pass it to others.

I invite my colleagues, indeed any of you in doubt, to look into my work, but do not ignore it. The suffering, of all human kind and of Nature (caused by human actions), is too severe. To continue on, because of ignorance, is simply irrational. Please, I urge you to hear this and reflect on my message!

I thank the many individuals who, directly and indirectly, have helped me better understand the various principles that have led me to the ideas expressed herein. You have my gratitude.

I am particularly grateful for the help, encouragement, and incredible patience I have received from Denise LaBee, a master listener and my editor, who never tried to subvert my determination or ideas and especially having to put up with my English, literally.

Special thanks to Steve Fargan for helping on the computer and organizing the index and Didi Chaney for the many final revisions to the manuscript and redoing the contents and the index.

To many people who encouraged me to write my book. My mentor Flo Collier, my dear friends Meili and Bob Murray, Henry (Tex) and Shirley Anderson, Paublo Trujillo, Diana, Dennis, Rachel and Birdie Overholser, Gina and Angela Sunshine, Michelle Nelson, Gene and Virginia Griswold, Eric and Vivica Henningsen, Ed & Peg Jensen, Lisa and Linda Goeringer, Zorica, Dragan and Marko Zivkovic, Vucko Antich, Doreen, Jake, Melody, Jasmine, Jenna, Gerri McManus, Sherry Bower Moore, Erica Hansen, Bill and Selma Marek, the Amadors, Halina, Stanly, Inga and Annaliza, Randy Johnson, Max Good and many others - thank you. My family, from whom I took the time to work on this project, a special, loving thanks. I cannot believe my patience and persistence in completing this work; thank you Nature God for assisting me.

Last but not least the Spirit Springs Foundation and my friend John Henningsen have been of a greatest help. I have always been encouraged in so many ways. He truly believes that everyone stands a greater chance to get healthier, regardless of age. Spirit Springs Foundation is a non-profit organization where I work with many people in need. The Foundation enables me to spread my knowledge to children, schools, and seniors - those who might otherwise not have access to the information. I want everyone to be more informed and aware of the cause of their problems. I am forever grateful that I can be of service in this way.

There is no such thing as a free lunch. In Nature, there are neither rewards nor punishments - only consequences. The **Cure** is in the **Cause**. We have to accept the Law of cause and effect or we will never find the cure. No technique exists that will cure anything on a permanent level if the cause is ignored. Today we are looking for symptoms, not the cause and because of it we have gone astray plugged with so-called incurable and degenerative diseases.

Nature's wisdom is life itself: health, happiness, harmony, love, success, and liberty. In these pages you will discover the simplicity of these eternal truths. You will never have to be ill.

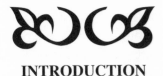

INTRODUCTION

Whenever a person wants to express his or her ideas, there always seems to be an important underlying cause - an awakening that made that person feel they have something to share.

I put this book together to help you understand better how and why we go through life experiences that sometimes feel impossible to bear. And yet we live through them, but with a desire to help others ease their pain, and our own.

I began this book long ago. It grew with me, I knew one day it would all come together when the time was right! My feelings deepened with time and life's experiences, with truths that revealed themselves, with the desperation of wanting answers and the why of life's consequences.

I must say it wasn't just me that was driving my burning desire, but rather a combination of many things, as you will see.

Along the way, I learned to be more patient and not to judge. I discovered that time truly *is* of the essence, and life experiences reveal to us an awareness that becomes a key able to unlock any door. Most of all, life is a bundle of causes and effects, our awareness and how we deal with it.

My entire life changed dramatically after nine years waiting for our first child's arrival. For the first time, I genuinely realized the true meaning of the words unconditional love, patience, sympathy, and deep sensitivity all in one. Pure love = truth!

Before we even brought our son home, I cried "mother's blues" wondering how anyone could have a child, a totally innocent being, and love him so much, then one day send him to war to get killed or kill some other innocent young man? The question struck me so hard I cried for days. I finally calmed down, but there was also something deeper in me that started to unfold.

I was never the same again. Instinctively I became more aware so I could greater protect his innocence. Questions that needed answers came from all directions. More naive then, many things slipped by without notice but the consequences were enormous. We do learn from our mistakes. If we don't learn the truth then we *will* repeat the mistakes again. I want to help you not to make the same mistakes.

Six short months after our son was born, we were told he had to be immunized. He was vaccinated with a combination injection that included a live polio virus. I vividly remember we had to sign a disclosure - the standard policy of hospitals and clinics. Our son became extremely ill. The doctors didn't know what to do other than say he'd had an allergic reaction to the vaccine. Then as now, there is no requirement to report allergic reactions to vaccines, but I will discuss immunizations and vaccines in depth later in the book.

All sorts of procedures were tried in an attempt to reduce the convulsions and tightness in our son's arms and legs. They wanted me to quit nursing him so he could stay in the hospital for a while. My instincts warned me not to stop nursing, nor to leave him alone in the hospital.

The next few years were the hardest of my life. Our son did not like or want to walk. They put braces on his legs day and night. A few months later, an orthopedic surgeon recommended tendon surgery to relieve the tightness in our son's legs. The procedure would have made him wheelchair bound for the rest of his life. That we could not do. I asked the doctor if he had a child like ours, would he allow the surgery? "Absolutely." That was too much to bear. We decided to seek alternatives and traveled to Europe. At the time, doctors there weren't recommending such radical procedures as a rule of thumb.

This time was difficult to live through. If it wasn't for a strong will to help an innocent child, prayer, and humility, I would not have been able to survive this rude awakening! But with hard work, persistence, a natural diet, exercise, and positive thinking, Nature (God) came to the rescue.

After changing my career to Alternative Medicine (Naturopathy) and learning more truth about health and life in general, I became more aware that there are many medical systems in the world that are in extreme conflict with one another. They all claim their fame, but look out! The one that does the least harm to the body with the least side effects should get the credit. Doctor Nature! Doctor means teacher in Latin. What have you learned from your doctor lately?

Many moons ago Dr. John Tilden said it so nicely that from time immemorial man has looked for savior, and when not looking for savior he's looking for cure. He's looking to get something for nothing, not knowing that the highest price we ever pay for anything is to have it given to us for free.

Instead of accepting salvation, it is better to deserve it. Instead of buying, begging to stealing a cure, it is better to stop building disease. Disease is of man's own building, and one worse thing than the stupidity of buying a cure is to remain so ignorant as to believe in cures without a cause.

The false theories of salvation and the cures have built man into a mental medicant – when he could be the arbiter of his own salvation and certainly his own doctor instead of being a slave to a profession that has neither worked out its own salvation from disease nor discovered a single cure in all the age long period of man's existence on earth.

We hear of diet cures, dieticians, balance rations, meat diets, blood type group diets, chemically prepared foods of all kinds. The reading and television public is bewildered with hundreds of health diet magazines and thousands of health ideas. Thousands are writing on health issues who would not recognize it if they should meet it on the street. Fanaticism, stupidity and commercialism are the principal elements in the dietetic industry that is belaboring the public. Cures are what the public want and cures are what the physicians and cultists affect to make; but at most only relief is given and unless the cause of toxemia is discovered (bad diet, habits and lifestyles) and removed, it will reoccur. The entire medical profession is engaged in treating crises of toxemia – curing? And curing? Until their patients are overtaken with chronic disease of whatever organ was the seat of the toxic crisis.

How many innocent children, adults and animals too, are the victims of wrongdoings: botched surgery, overdoses, incorrect prescriptions, and allergic reactions? No one outside the medical establishment knows for certain. That information is not available to us, as we will discover later on.

Bertrand Russell said that *Man's half-cleverness would be the means of his own destruction.* Going against Nature will destroy us.

Cancer alone kills more than five hundred thousand Americans, and 2.2 billion dollars of taxpayers' money is spent on cancer research every year. Can you imagine what else we could do with 2.2 billion dollars if everyone could read the truth about cancer's true cause? Cancer's cause is known, as are the causes of other degenerative diseases. Why is the truth hidden? Read on and stay open-minded.

There is incredible harm done on the misinformed and frightened patients. They are literally paying with their lives. The scars are immense, visible, man-made damage, yet there is far more damage that we cannot see. Consequences are surfacing and are shocking. Incorrect facts or their interpretation unchallenged, become mistakenly accepted as the truth. When false facts are mixed among the real facts, confusion is inevitable leading to more mistakes and misunderstanding over the real cause. In order to realize the truth, the false information must be identified and the true information must be put together and brought to light so it can be seen and heard by the ones that proved it to themselves and can do the same for all others. Many times this is very difficult because our hands are tied from the opposing side that does not want the truth to be heard or seen and will do anything to stop it.

You will see in the pages ahead that society's survival has always depended on unconventional ways of thinking. According to conventional wisdom this persecution "protects the public" but in reality it harms them and impedes progress. Suppression keeps the real truth from surfacing and protects the economic interest of the status quo.

Modern medicine wants to talk about statistics and scientific research. I do not want to be a statistic and neither should you. Statistics can be manipulated to suit the viewpoint of the person quoting them. Numbers can be skewed due to a variety of circumstances like heredity, nutrition, or lifestyle. Statistics are a tool, not a fact.

The fact is that the cure of any problem or disease is in the cause. So in reality we know the cure; we just cannot comprehend it. Therefore, we do not think about removing the cause, not even trying to analyze possible reasons, we bury it deeper by treating the symptoms. The **Cure** is in the **Cause**.

You will also see that in order to cure a person of any health problem, it has to begin with that person's **awareness of their problem, the cause and changing their out look on health and life**. You must look inward and find balanced awareness. The mind is the major influence on the body and freedom from disease depends upon connection of our own awareness to bring the balance and to extend that harmony throughout the body. Nutrition is the key, real key, since the *brain* in order to keep harmony, also needs certain nutrients.

You will come to peace with this understanding of mind, body, emotion and spirit as we move along. The pieces of the puzzle will all fall into place. They did for me when I finally came to peace with it all.

One day my son and I were walking leisurely on a beach in Oregon. It was a beautiful summer day and the timing was just right. Suddenly we looked at each other without a word. We both wanted to say something but nothing was coming out. I could see peace on his face and I finally started to apologize to him about all the terrible things that we had to go through, thinking that we were doing him good. He just listened. With tears in my eyes, finally spilling my wounded heart out to him, I wanted him to know that it was irresponsibility, ignorance and lack of research. I did not know the horrible consequences of my decision and allowing this to happen. I am guilty and am so sorry. He was trying to stop me from talking and nodding his head while I continued on. How could Nature have rewarded me with such a perfectly innocent human being, and what right did I have to let the doctors and nurses decide what was best for you.

He grabbed my hand and with total peace and in a warm-sounding voice whispered to me:

"Mama, just listen to me for a moment. I have no hard feelings, grudges, and have forgiven everyone. I am fine now.

Whatever happened to me is history and you will see to it that it never happens again to other children. Tell all the parents the truth about vaccines, health, raw food, and all the other things you learned. Don't charge the children who come to see you. Nobody can ever stop you then."

I could not believe the words coming out of this young man. We slowly resumed our walk but I was never the same again. His words ring in my heart every time I see a child, and I've never charged children for a consultation. With this enormous message an urge to tell the truth became so strong that I no longer could stop, or be stopped regardless of what might happen to me.

For my son, all the kids and people in the world that suffer needlessly, I devote my life. I am blessed and grateful to be of help. I search for truth that is in us, and all around us. Sometimes we just miss it because we don't see it and feel it. We have been taught to ignore it. Because we do not look to the cause, we cannot find the answer - **The Cure.**

"The gold comes to the place where the injury was and is . . . I find this idea to be a truly amazing concept. I mean, the idea that the human beings wound and genius are located at the same place. It is from this spot where we are wounded that we will give our main gift to the community and the world."
Robert Bly

It was from this wound to my son, and by extension to my mother's soul, that the gold of my career change to Natural healing sprang.

The truths that I talk about are not man made and because of that, they have to be obeyed even more if you are to get better and resolve your life problems. You have to stick with the permanent laws of Nature that never change. We must keep an eye on the **Cause**.

Obedience to Nature's Wisdom equals life itself: health, happiness, harmony, love, success and liberty. They are all one and an inseparable truth. If you miss one, you will be out of balance and out of harmony. You have to go back and see where you have strayed away from Nature. This is the only reliable truth, each complete in harmony with each other and the universal laws of cause and effect. For every action, there is a reaction.

This book contains separate chapters for each of the simple truths about life. Included are many true stories from different people and their circumstances that show you how they got better when they took Nature's path and responsibility for their own health.

The laws of Nature are permanent. They will apply now and for eternity. By trusting in eternal truth you will always be on the right path - Nature's path. For this simple reason, this book will never be outdated.

This is not a new idea, cult or a new fad, so nothing has changed. This is the truth about permanent, eternal and forever laws of Nature that have been overlooked. Disastrous consequences are occurring as a result. If it sounds too simple to be true, don't step over it lightly. Please be open, become once and for all in touch with the inner universal consciousness that is in you and all of us.

We can only heal and be healed when we go back to Nature. We have no time to waste. Time is of the essence. When you are at peace with yourself and the world, you are one with Nature and Nature is one with you. Listen to your true guide and you will see all your problems vanish (physical, mental, emotional and spiritual).

For every problem, there are many solutions; in fact if it weren't for the solutions, the problem would not even exist. We are no longer capable of thinking as clearly. We no longer know what is wrong and what is right. This trend reminds me of the Roman Empire, and the ups and downs of all civilizations.

Earth and its habitat have been around for a long, long time. Humans were the last to arrive and perhaps we must be the first to leave in order to cure the planet Earth and its habitat of our enormous damage that we caused and continue to cause. *"The meek shall inherit the earth."*

We have managed just fine for centuries obeying our instinctive nature, getting by and could have continued for eternity. Something went wrong, especially the last hundred years. We stopped obeying nature's most important law: **the Law of Cause**

and Effect and we are paying enormous consequences as you will see ahead.

I will show you how this can all be reversed. Knowing this simple truth, what caused our problems can cure us by stopping it/eliminating it, regardless of what it is. I urge you now to reflect on this.

You will find out in the pages ahead that I'm not trying to be right or act arrogantly or smart. I just see it and feel it. The answers are always simple. You don't have to be a genius. You only have to be aware of what goes on around you. Consequences are here now.

Many times laws that are man-made sooner or later become obsolete, broken, changed, or diverted to fit the masses and certain special-interest groups. Then new groups come along and change the laws to fit themselves, so previous laws become invalid. The laws will change again and again. None work for long if at all and certainly not for you. How can they if they are not in accordance with Nature? Nature's laws are not prejudicial; they work for everyone, regardless. They are eternal.

In the pages ahead you will see why doctors don't live very long, why they suffer from many different diseases and why *they* come to alternative doctors for help. They are truly not trained to think on purpose. Their reluctance is often linked to their reliance on "scientific proof." Many doctors are trained to memorize facts and statistics. If they were interested in true healing, medical schools would make nutrition a mandatory and integral part of their learning. They prescribe drugs that treat your symptoms. To make things worse they are not even aware of this but that's where the money is, not in teaching patients to change their diet and lifestyle. In many cases modern medical thinking leaves the patient in worse condition than before they saw the doctor.

The real reason why most doctors *do not believe* that nutrition has anything to do with ill health is that the food we eat today is *highly processed*, laden with pesticides, growth hormones, artificial flavors and preservatives that actually cause ill health and disease. If we ate live, raw, fresh food and herbs in their original form, it would heal and repair damaged organs and doctors would prescribe this to their patients. For some strange reason they have missed this simple truth. That's where the answers lie.

However out of over one hundred twenty-nine universities that teach medicine, only twenty-nine offer nutritional courses. Even then the courses are not made mandatory. Doctors do not take these courses on their own because the ones who pay their scholarships discourage nutrition. Mandatory nutrition courses are taught in only a very few universities. Even then the nutrition they teach is not true nutrition.

The biggest, most dangerous threat to all mankind and our planet comes from the destroyers - subtle and unseen - the poisons of our water, soil and the degeneration of our food and environment.

Before school I was taught to be responsible for the things I do and for the things that I do not do. Unfortunately, this is not taught in many homes, schools and especially in medical schools.

You will see in the pages ahead that there is no such thing as incurable disease. Maybe an incurable patient (as Dr. Bernard Jensen told) is one that does not want to change his/her bad habits and follow natural laws. The price will be the accumulation of plaque, toxins, chemicals and inorganic matter that will cause all sorts of disease, ill health and disharmony.

Find out how any problem, with just a little common sense, can be alleviated, avoided and should never be tolerated by intelligent people.

Let's bring our awareness up so that we can live a lot longer, happier for many years to come and without suffering. We can, so long as we stay on Nature's path. She provides answers when science fails anxiously warning, calling us again and again to listen to her beat of the drum.

So let's respond right now with the beginning and life itself.

Best regards,

R. B.

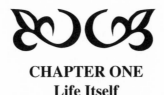

CHAPTER ONE
Life Itself

"Inconceivable as it may seem to ordinary reason, you and all other conscious beings as such are all in all. Hence this life of yours which you are living is not merely a piece of the entire existence, but is in a certain sense the whole."
Erwin Schroedinger, *My View Of The World*

Life always was, is, and will remain a mystery.

Life itself is a vibrational energy behind Nature's forces that gives life to the universe, solar systems, and earth. In harmony it connects us all. Laws of cause and effect. Action and reaction, gravity, supply and demand, etc.

The primal laws of cause and effect have no exceptions. The laws are always happening, automatically, forever and ever, physical, mental, emotional and spiritual all in one.

Life is energy and matter in motion. Life constantly arises from a source, and returns to that source. All life is energy in motion, and Nature (God) is the source. All movement flows from positive through neutral to negative and back again cyclically. The cycles in our daily lives are fascinating to observe. Day, night, birth, life, death. Winter, spring, summer, fall. Everything that surrounds us goes through constant changes, like the ebb and flow of tides, or phases of the moon. See how we are in tune with the source? This is a permanent law.

The universe is made up of one kind of entity. Each one is alive; each determines the course of its own existence. Don't worry - even death is alive! We are all equal beings. We are kin to the universe and everything that surrounds us. Cause and effect, expansions and contraction, action and reaction, balance and imbalance, yin and yang.

Each entity is a duplication of Nature, some universal force, or God, as you prefer. The explanation truly does not matter. We exist and the universe exists. However, in order for us to exist in tune with this incredible entity, we must obey Nature, without a doubt, or pay the consequences. Life is well-controlled and organized to function automatically according to Nature's laws, just as our subconscious mind handles the very complicated functions of our body without us knowing or thinking about it.

"May we say that the soul has been forever in a state of knowledge? And if the truth about reality is always in our soul, the soul must be immortal, and one must take courage and try to discover - that is, to recollect what one doesn't happen to know or (more correctly) remember, at the moment."

Socrates

Unless we follow the laws of Nature we cannot escape the problems. Again, the infallible law of cause and effect, along with our thoughts and feelings, are the most powerful conditions in our daily lives.

History repeats itself. The mistakes of the past receive only temporary notice and they are repeated over and over again. Some dangerous mistakes and errors are responsible for our current health problems and their severity. They seem to become more evident now and are the result of human over-confidence and obsession of science and technology yet complete ignorance of the fundamental laws of Nature-simple truth. Things are desperate. The writing is on the wall and our future is in jeopardy.

Mankind has strayed from this simple wisdom and these basic laws, causing us to experience all sorts of trouble and problems we cannot see or feel. Who knows what would it take to turn things around? In some cases and some areas of our existence, is it perhaps too late? One thing is certain; it will take us going back to Nature to find true answers to all our problems.

Even though false knowledge is far more dangerous than

ignorance, we are surrounded by both. Thankfully, we have the choice to see things in a truthful way. It's not always easy.

Can you imagine if people still believed that the Earth was flat? What if we knew differently and could prove it? We would be punished. Most all believe that germs are our enemies. We can prove that they are not, but we sometimes get punished for that and suffer endlessly.

Today we have new technology, new information. Plainly we've been around for a while, but we are still in the dark about many things. Truth is sometimes hidden from us intentionally. Lies are taught to us constantly. We cannot even detect them any longer. Lies become truth to us because we have gotten confused for many generations. Truth is buried from us. If you are not determined to get to the bottom of it all you will struggle needlessly all your life. We must remain open-minded because change is permanent. New discoveries bring new theories that seem to make more sense to us, yet later they may be replaced by other theories that again make no sense.

"Physicists have come to see that all their theories of natural phenomena, including the laws they describe, are creations of human mind . . . The physicist begins his inquiry into the essential nature of things by studying the material world. Penetrating even deeper realms of matter, he has become aware of the essential unity of all things and events. More than that, he has also learned that he himself, and his consciousness, are an integral part of this unity."
Fritjof Capra

From **Deepak Chopra**, *Infinite Possibilities:*

Understanding the Quantum Mechanical Human Body:

"Physics informs us that the basic fabric of nature lies at the quantum level, far beyond atoms and molecules. A quantum, defined as the basic unit of matter or energy, is from 10 million to 100 million times smaller than the smallest atom. At this level, matter and energy become interchangeable. All quanta are made of invisible vibrations - ghosts of energy - waiting to take physical form. The same is true of the human body - it first takes form as intense but invisible vibrations, called quantum fluctuations, before it proceeds to coalesce into impulses of energy - and particles of matter.

"At the quantum level, no part of the body lives apart from the rest. There are no wires holding together the molecules of your arteries, just as there are no visible connections binding together the stars in the galaxy. Yet arteries and galaxies are both securely held together, in a seamless perfect design. The invisible bonds that you cannot examine under microscope are quantum in nature; without this 'hidden physiology', your visible physiology could not exist. It would never have been more than a random collection of molecules.

"The only way to truly penetrate this realm is subjectively from inside the quantum mechanical body. Here is where the trick of turning mind into matter is actually being managed. Your mind gives you control, the ability to have any reaction you want. The great misfortune is that all of us are preprogrammed along extremely rigid lines; we have only a few reactions instead of infinite ones. Because of that, we pay a price. The mind-body connection ceases to be effortless and natural; stress starts to accumulate, and negative signals from the mind begin to damage the cells. An old Indian saying goes: "If you want to see what your thoughts were yesterday, look at your body today. If you want to see what your body will be like tomorrow, look at your thoughts today." *The real medicine our body needs is medicine for our awareness. Once you know that there is a quantum body*

paralleling your physical one, many things make sense that were mysteries before.

"Getting back in touch with the quantum mechanical body is the most important goal in Ayurveda. We call this process 'quantum healing'. As understood by modern medicine, the body's healing abilities are nearly infinite, but quantum healing is infinite. The flow of intelligence bubbling up from the quantum mechanical body can be channeled in countless ways to achieve any results in the physical body, including the cure of serious, life-threatening diseases and the reversal of the aging process itself.

"Everything we think and do originates inside the quantum mechanical body and then bubbles up to the surface of life. You are not an isolated organism in time and space, occupying six cubic feet of volume and lasting seven or eight decades. Rather you are one cell in the cosmic body, entitled to all the privileges of your cosmic status, including perfect health. Nature made us thinking so that we could realize this truth. The inner intelligence of the body is the ultimate and supreme genius in nature. It mirrors the wisdom of the cosmos. This genius is the inside of you, a part of your inner blueprint that cannot be erased."

Again, it remains that life is such that we have to obey Nature's laws in order to live in harmony with the Universal laws. Every particle in every atom is a live being. Every molecule or cell is a tribe of beings. Energy is vibration. We can trust the flow of the universe - God.

It certainly makes us feel good to know these simple truths about life. You do not need to worry any more about your problems or fear anything knowing that every solution is in the cause. So every problem has a solution. In fact, many solutions. You will achieve total peace and tranquility about one and all. You are in control of your destiny. We can revert back to the cause of any possible problem and be able to identify it without any difficulties. Can it possibly get any simpler than that?

Let's look into the possibilities of where we came from and the natural ways of life and nutrition to harmonize our biological, physical body.

Origins

"*Humans are made up of a procession of phantoms, in the midst of which there strides an unknowable reality.*"
Dr. Alexis Carrel, *Man The Unknown*

We are created by Nature (God). There are so many great questions for which we have no answers. So many theories, including Darwin's evolution theory, aren't quite right as we once thought.

Who knows the real answer about our origin? We often can't say with certainty what happened a minute ago. How can we claim to know what occurred one hundred thousand or one million years in the past? We can't. And that's why theories remain only speculation.

There are some interesting contradictions about the current theories of evolution, the supportive fossil records (or lack thereof), the true definition of what a species is, random mutations, genetics, natural selection, embryology, diet, science and philosophy of our origins that beg further dialogue and research. There really isn't room to do the subject justice here, but an excellent place to start is *Darwin on Trial*, by Phillip Johnson.

Growing up, I often wondered about evolution, but when I wanted to talk further with my high school biology teacher about Darwin's theory, she kicked me out of class. Looking back, I realize she felt threatened because she probably didn't have any answers that weren't in the standard textbook. Since then, I've done my own learning and discovered that Darwin himself, in *Descent of Man*, admitted his oversight in failing to consider the existence of many structures that appear to be neither beneficial nor injurious to the origin of species as a part of natural selection.

I feel safe to say that Homo Sapiens are an outcome of some Incomprehensible Intelligence. Physically and biologically, humans are one of the most incredibly organized living machines ever constructed by efforts of Nature - God. We are as strong as our weakest link, and natural selection takes care of its own strength. No technology could ever surpass the magnificence of our own biological design.

Nature literally performs miracles. Nature is just.

We will see that our true nature is biologically fruitarian; in other words, we are primarily eaters of fruits, herbs, along with green leafy vegetables, seeds and nuts. There is a reason for this.

It's very important to know that originally humans were mainly fruit and herb eaters. Our weaknesses today are due to the fact we eat too much meat and processed food, only some fruit and a few empty inorganic vegetables. On top of that, we ruin the good foods we do eat by cooking them, which changes their chemical structure and destroys natural enzymes. Our body must work hard to convert cooked food so it can be utilized to some extent - with a high price to pay in the form of depletion of the enzymes our body stores in case of emergency. It's passed crisis level a long time ago. This is where our problems lie today. We are now born lacking important enzymes and wonder why we are degenerated, even as children. Before we are even born! Pancreatic disorder and cancer are becoming among the number one leading causes of death.

No new technology could ever surpass the incredible magnificence of our own biological design. But man-made habits can take it away from us. It took a long time to get where we are, yet we've managed to ruin it so quickly. We need to think more about this. Reversal will take a long time, if it can be done at all.

Many of my colleagues are concerned and wonder if we have not gone past the point of no return.

Interfering with Nature isn't good, but when we go against her, that's where our problems are difficult to turn around. The damage is done in so many ways we aren't even aware of any more. We ignore it completely. Consequences are here now. What are we going to do about it and when?

GEF (genetically engineered food) and GMO (genetically modified organism) contain altered cell information the result of artificially transferring genes from one species to another by first identifying a gene with desired trait from a plant, animal or bacterium. The gene is then isolated and removed, then injected in the bacterial cell that copies it millions of times over and ferries it into a target organism. Genes too can be injected into a target organism without being multiplied using a particle gun. Then Nature weaves the protein string into a new strand of DNA. The trouble is when a target cell takes up the inserted gene, it could end up anywhere. The gene may attach in the middle of another gene and totally interfere with the normal function of that cell. It could damage the DNA of the host that will lead to food that contains allergens and toxins with unknown health effects. Have you heard of people allergic to nuts because they are allergic to soybeans engineered to contain a protein from brazil nuts? Once GMO cross-pollinates with wild counterparts and weeds, there is no way to stop it. Pollen dispersal from GE crops has been recorded at up to three kilometers by air flow and four kilometers by insects. Mike Ligiori, Communications Coordinator for Citizens for Health (which is in charge of GMO labeling), says: "Fundamental and irreversible changes are being made in the food supply. The long term effects are unprecedented and unknown and there is no thought put into it."

When I was on sabbatical in New Zealand (New Zealand is one of the first countries in the world to use GMO and GEF) I realized for the first time what incredible damage had been done to all life and I believe that the problem of GMOs in a few years would not be able to revert to the cause due to its multiplicity and because it is out of control. Why should people pay the price of scientific research with their lives and future uncertainties.

Cornell University researchers found that pollen from GE corn can kill Monarch butterfly larvae. Half of the summer the Monarch population is concentrated in the U.S. cornbelt. Monarchs are at much at risk from habitat destruction in Mexico where they reside in winter. Within a few years all traditional food crops will be contaminated with GMOs and we may not have pure food seeds to grow. Since we are responsible for the things that we do as well as for the things that we do not do, we have to become aware of the consequences. Seek organic non-hybridized seeds.

GE is not a natural extension of traditional cross-breeding. It is common knowledge that in traditional cross-breeding or hybridization, Nature will only allow the mixing of genes from the same or closely related species. GE allows scientists to completely ignore the natural reproductive boundaries established over billions of years. Instead, through invasive viruses or instruments like gene guns, the DNA from completely unrelated organisms - like fish and strawberries, bacteria and soybeans, or humans and pigs - can be intermingled. What's worse is the technology itself is imprecise, uncontrolled and random. When we insert genes that would not naturally be a part of a living organism, we will have the cause of unexpected consequences - consequences for the organism being modified, the ecosystem of which that organism is a part and for the people consuming some or all of that organism as food.

"Life does not occur without life. Every part of the body is dependent on the whole."

"Nature and evolution dislike waste and whenever possible they use tissues for other purposes when the type of structure and form of life change. The only permanent thing in life is change."

"Nothing endures unless it is of use in the world and in the economy of Nature."

"Civilized man does not add to the beauties of Nature, but generally destroys, prevents, or disarranges the progress of natural changes."

Dr. Charles Mayo

Let's just look at a few examples in respect to our immune system and the antibiotic tragedy.

Immune System Problems

People will perish due to lack of knowledge and unawareness.

Threats to our immune system are on the rise. Despite technology and modern medicine, we live in an age that presents staggering risks to our body's built-in defense mechanisms.

Today microbes and viruses can affect us differently than they used to because of our general weakening. Our bodies are overloaded with debris. Tuberculosis is back and spreading because drugs-antibiotics have made us weaker. Many other "new" viruses, Hepatitis A, B and C for example, are on the rise for the same reason, too. The increased amounts of free radicals (cancer-causing agents) and growth hormones in the dairy foods we're exposed to cause uncontrolled cellular growth and suppressed immunity. I'll talk about cellular-level problems later on. Suffice it to say we have become weaker than our ancestors.

The miracle drugs of yesterday are nearly useless today against many strains of bacteria and antibiotics have caused the suppression of symptoms by driving the disease deeper into the tissue that later creates more problems and illness. Bacteria are the same as always. We are not. We have to pay the price now for becoming too dependent on antibiotics to knock out drug-resistant bugs that our immune system can't handle. Antibiotics have also invaded our food supply. Animals are routinely given massive doses of drugs to get rid of infections due to poor immune systems. Antibacterial products - hand soaps, dishwashing liquids, countertop scrubs, toilet bowl cleansers, body washes, etc. - have flooded the market, creating new strains of bacteria by their indiscriminate overuse. This makes us more stressed and weaker.

Antibiotics destroy both good and bad bacteria in the colon and increase the risk of opportunistic infections like Candida (yeast), that move in when normal intestinal flora have been eliminated - wiped out by antibiotics. Our body was not designed to be treated with artificial inputs, so we have to pay with enormous consequences. Weakened immune systems.

Sadly, we do not appreciate our immune system. We abused it until it no longer functions properly. Our immune system contains three types of white blood cells: 1) natural killer cells, 2) the B cells that produce antibodies, and 3) the specialized T cells that target and kill microbes. Scientists have uncovered a group of chemical messengers that different cells of the immune system use to communicate with each other: beneficial T cells, helper T cells that react to a foreign invader and start the immune reaction, killer T cells which directly attack infectious agents, and suppresser T cells that turn off the immune reaction once the infection has been conquered. Out defense system cannot communicate properly with drugs.

Just look what we have done by depending on antibiotics. Impaired immune system function will continue out of control, but we will have new names for it.

While aging immune systems weaken, some become overactive, leading to an increase in auto-immune reactions. In that case, immune cells target and destroy the body's own cells by mistakenly perceiving them as foreign intruders or enemies.

What are the consequences? We have no clue how well our immune system works until we have a cold or come down with the flu. In fact, it's always working and active, even when you're asleep, patrolling the blood stream to scour out any foreign bacteria or virus, and destroying pre-cancerous cells.

When your system is weakened, you are much more susceptible to virtually every type of illness. Remember, **there is no disease without a weak body**. The immune system is critical to your body's self-healing mechanism, whether it's healing a little bruise, or recovering from surgery or long illness.

You can also become ill as a result of an overly active immune system. Many auto-immune disorders - rheumatoid arthritis, pernicious anemia, chronic thyroiditis, lupus, multiple sclerosis - are linked to inappropriate or self-attacking immune system activity.

For instance, in rheumatoid arthritis, the immune cells mistakenly target the body's own tissue, resulting in painful inflammation and gradual deterioration of cartilage. Instead of cleansing and strengthening the body, pain medications are prescribed to lessen the symptoms.

This is all related to a confused mind/body to the point that we do not function with chemical correctness to certain impulses that are sent from the brain into the body's organs and glands.

This is why it is so difficult to help people with multiple illnesses without looking to the real cause-the originator of the problem. It all goes back to the root of the problems that are very much related to what we put in our body so we can function in harmony within.

The key now is how to boost, balance and strengthen our immune system.

It is very crucial here that we get to the '**root of the roots**.' Everything counts. Don't let anybody fool you on this point. Our immune system didn't go off-kilter all of a sudden. It started with childhood vaccines (more later on *that* sore subject), and intensified with tonsillectomies, appendectomies, antibiotics for minor ear infections, gall bladder removals, kidney stones, and hysterectomies, to name a few. And this is where we are today; stuck with diseases we've created. Surprised? Just look at what we've eaten the last fifty years - frozen dinners, powdered milk, canned vegetables, preservatives, sodium nitrate, meals in a box, and meals in plastic. And the plague of our society: high-fat fast foods that skip every important nutrient group.

We need to improve our bodily systems by first eliminating all the burdens of today's temporary-fix solution - suppression of symptoms with drugs. Then start from scratch by identifying and correcting the underlying cause of illness (healing); detecting problems early, before symptoms or disease develop (prevention); helping to determine if your health program is working (feedback); and optimizing health and promoting longevity (wellness).

Before any of this, we must:

1) Clean out the elimination channels (bowel, skin, lungs and lymph system, etc.).
2) Flush out the toxic settlements (by fasting and eating only natural food).
3) Supply the body with proper and balanced nutrients (organic, raw food).

Once this program is in place you will not be able to find disease. When you do the right thing, you can expect the right results. Truth is simple. Look deep, as Dr. Bernard Jensen teaches.

We have to realize that many health professionals look at and treat symptoms, not the cause. Whatever the reason, old-fashioned tests like pH, tissue, urine or hair sample analysis, and remedies like good food, fresh air, sun, and laughter are often ignored today. Are they too simple for the "constipated profession"?

Again, I bring up Dr. Bernard Jensen and his simple truth. Let the elimination process discharge and get rid of catarrh (debris-carrying mucus). The worst thing we can do is to stop mucus (runny nose, cough, temperature) by taking drugs. We build the disease. Bacteria like weak tissue (it cannot survive without it). Any organ that overworks burns off the natural sodium and weakens. Eat all natural foods - variety is the key - that way we store minerals in the body. Then when we need them our body will be able to use them.

Approximately eighty-five percent of people have chronic diseases and are only being treated for the symptoms they exhibit. Every disease is a sign of a chemical shortage or imbalance of some sort, if it's under-active or overworking.

Don't heat oils or fry your food. Take care of the bowel and toxic material. Let everything keep coming and going. Don't stop anything artificially. Ask yourself: is it natural, is it pure, is it whole? If it doesn't spoil, it's not natural or any good. Look for the **Cause** of your symptom. That's where the cure is too.

We know now what to do and what not to do. Nature's way is *the* way, even if you have to go alone, but we must return to where the problem originated in order to find a key. Wisdom is the ability to discover an alternative and to look for solutions.

For instance, vaccination is a highly controversial subject. Vaccinations are needless and may be very dangerous, in a short and long run. Many cases of polio and small pox were the results of vaccinations. The DPT has also been shown to have detrimental effects in some children. Many times we do not know the damage until later in life (breaking down of immune system, regression in development and many physical and mental disabilities that are so difficult to trace). The structure of vaccines is such that there is no doubt that illness could be triggered later by the use of vaccines.

The new vaccines claim to prevent harmful diseases. Even if they did, the risk is greater in the long and short run. If a child contracts these diseases, they could be treated correctly - naturally, the illness is not life threatening. When a child is raised properly he would not contract any disease to begin with. There is no disease in a healthy body that is free of mucus and antibiotic damage. The body's cellular environment is the key.

Please read <u>Murder by Injection</u> and <u>The Poisoned Needle</u>. Write:

National Health Federation
P.O. Box 688
Monrovia, CA 91017

There will be more on this subject later. Be sure to inform yourself so you don't make the mistakes many and I did.

The number one key is to keep the blood clean of mucus by eating fresh food the way Nature provided. Staying on Nature's path.

More than anything, the greatest contribution we can make for the new generation is to prepare them to think for themselves, so they can become aware of the truth and Nature's immutable laws.

How to live in harmony with Nature
Taking a fresh look at a new you

"Every morning was a cheerful invitation to make my life of equal simplicity and I may say innocence with Nature herself."
Henry David Thoreau

"Come forth into the light of things, let nature be your teacher. Nature never did betray the heart that loved her."
William Wordsworth

"Love all God's creation, both the whole and every grain of sand. Love every leaf, every ray of light. Love the animals, love the plants, love each separate thing. If thou love each thing thou wilt perceive the mystery of God in all; and when once thou perceive this, thou wilt thenceforth grow every day to a fuller understanding of it: until thou come at last to live the whole world with love that will then be all-embracing and universal."
Dostoevsky

Some of us like myself were lucky enough to grow up living in tune with Nature. We planted our food, lived somewhat primitively - no electricity or running water, no processed food, no car, phone, TV, VCR, or any of today's modern technology. I believe we were also happier and more content. We were stronger physically and mentally. Instinctively we were survivors in cases of man-made or natural disasters. Today we are being raised where we have everything on a silver platter. Our instincts are weaker and we misjudge the real truth. But we cannot blame new technology for everything. It has given us so much and outwardly, life seems easier now. However, when you look back and really compare the past with the present, you will realize we gave up a lot to obtain what we have now. We may have to give up even more, for the new millennium is ahead with yet more technology and "simpler" living. But remember, there will be a greater price to pay. There is no free lunch. The only free cheese is in a mousetrap.

When we physically worked harder, our lives were simpler and we appreciated and enjoyed things more because of it. I *feel* this.

I was raised with the changing of seasons, and Nature was truly my teacher. My family prepared for every season and were in turn always rewarded for staying in tune with Nature. *"As you sow, so shall you reap."* Literally. This was a way of life for us. When the rewards came we truly enjoyed them, shared them, and humbly thanked Nature by giving it all back to the soil. Heaven on Earth, I thought, until my grandmother told me Heaven was even better! I couldn't believe that anything like that could even be possible.

Today we have all the modern conveniences of life and not enough time to push all the buttons, much less watch a flower open or listen to sweet birdsong. We can still choose, and hope that we will always be able to choose. The choices we make today are often less in tune with Nature. The price may be higher, the trade-offs greater, but we are in charge. The one constant in life is that things will change, and we have to keep up with the changes and yet stay in tune with Nature.

We are in the drastic revisions of transition. Every aspect of our society is changing: politics, medicine, education, economics, religion, workplace, and family. Are things changing for the better? We all hope so. One thing is certain, we must have our roots fixed deeper in Nature to survive the transitions. This is where our balance and harmony will make us feel secure, no matter how drastic our life changes.

Somehow we must stay in touch with the divine and let the moment-to-moment enjoyment of simplicity and that magnificent power of eternity and satisfaction toy with us. To oblige ourselves to Nature's laws that are permanent, regardless of time; to live without leaving any hour behind; to be frugal and not waste natural resources; to use only what we need; to give more than to take; and, to listen deep inside where all the answers are. To live simply and in tune with Nature's majesty so that we can become aware of the real truth.

> *"To take what there is, and use it, without waiting forever in vain for the preconceived - to dig deep into the actual and get something out of that truth - this doubtless is the right way to live."*
>
> **Henry James**

I am very excited about the new millennium and all the changes for the betterment of humanity. I feel deep inside that more and more we want to know the truth and the cause of everything. If not now, when? We have the technology to wipe out all the dogma by pushing the right button on the computer and sending everyone a message of truth. It sounds farfetched, but I truly believe when true knowledge is given to young children from the very beginning, it's like a sunflower that turns its blossom automatically toward the brightest, purest source of light. That's where our Nature is, always knowing what's right. It's inborn in all of us. We've just been misguided unknowingly and have been in trouble for it in all aspects of our lives.

Now that we know why and where we went astray, we have a steppingstone to take it a bit further, wider, higher, and most of all kindlier, so that we do not have to make others suffer. Then we too will have peace.

We have to understand the importance that life does not occur without life. So to think that some scientific intervention is necessary is not a permanent fix but rather a quick fix with consequences down the road. We need to understand this, for instance bacteria is necessary for life as a minute chemist of the air, water and soil. Bacteria are our friends. We need them. Germs and viruses have taken the spot light in the fight against disease. Yet they are not the real cause of the disease as you will find out.

We would not have to worry so much about curing a disease if we know what caused it. We would prevent it then from happening in the first place. So today's progress – the means of relief by drugs or surgery has outstripped our knowledge of the cause of disease. We have gotten blinded by medical progress. Very few are interested in knowing the cause and how we ever allowed it to go this far is incredible.

Modern agriculture, with all its subcultures, has its foundation in evolution. It does *not* seek to understand the soil-plant relation from the Creator's standpoint, by reasoning from cause to effect in husbanding the soil. Rather, it must wait for disease to show itself. It then names the symptoms and attacks the symptoms with substances that are usually foreign and poisonous to the biologic systems of plants, animals, and humans.

Many organic and eco-ag. approaches have also clung to the basic concepts of modern agriculture and still work on the symptoms, although with less harmful substances. Because the root cause of many soil and plant problems are the same, it becomes a trial and error or a gambling approach to find the solution. Like all gambling, a very few win, while most do not.

Dr. A. F. Beddoe

Staying in balances with nature and taking good care of our soil is the key to our future survival. If the plant is not nourished with the proper elements that are in the soil, food will be depleted and our body will degenerate. Please look into Dr. Beddoe's book on soil: Nourishment Home Grown.

The following is an Indian Ute prayer, given to me by my friend and assistant Michele Nelson. The kindness and love she shares and gives to many needy people and animals is simply incredible. I wept upon reading this. Thank you to the one who created this beautiful poem.

Earth Prayer

Earth teach me stillness as the grass is stilled with light.
Earth teach me suffering, as old stone suffers with memory.
Earth teach me humility as blossoms are humble with beginning.
Earth teach me caring, as the mother who secures her young.
Earth teach me courage as the tree which stands above.
Earth teach me limitation as the ant which crawls on the ground.
Earth teach me freedom as the eagle which soars in the sky.
Earth teach me respiration as the leaves which die in the fall.
Earth teach me regeneration as the seed which rises in the spring.
Earth teach me to forget myself as melted snow forgets its life.
Earth teach me to remember kindness as dry fields weep with rain.

Why is the Cure always in the Cause?

In America, it is against the law to treat cancer naturally in a way that eliminates the cause. On the contrary, the standard medical treatments contribute even further to the destruction of these valuable organs. Highly effective cancer therapies are illegal in the United States. When we understand the true cause, we also understand the proper treatment. But to admit true cause compels, true solution and there isn't any profit in it for the medical industry.

The disease is never acquired. It is always earned. Disease is a natural result obtained from unnatural lifestyle. Disease is not a question of exposure. It is an internal development which can lead to exposure susceptibility (environment).

Disease occurs only when one's internal environment is favorable for disease growth. We create our internal environment, yet we have been programmed to believe that people are constantly "catching" the flu, a bug or a virus from someone else. The truth is that ninety-nine percent has been creating a polluted internal environment capable of catching or creating any disease.

Being a doctor does not endow one with extraordinary knowledge of a cure if that doctor is not looking for a cause. They are not trained in medical schools to look for the cure. Rather, too much attention is given to developing the memory and too little to developing the mind. Too much stress is put on acquiring knowledge and not on the wise application of knowledge.

Every part of the body is dependent on the whole and what constitutes health is the key. Prevention is the most important factor. Medical progress and surgery have outstripped our knowledge of the disease and what causes it.

Take a look at this simple analogy and how Nature's law of **cause and effect** applies to all of us. Always, forever, without exception.

You have been getting a flat tire on the way to work over and over again. You take it in and fix it but it happens again. Your "bad luck" is getting worse and you're beginning to wonder who to blame: the tire mechanic, manufacturer, the car, even the road that you drive on. You even take another road to work and yet you have another flat tire. This is it. Somebody is out to get you. For the last time you take it in to have it fixed and you notice that your neighbor is there too. He has also had several flat tires lately and thought that someone was out to get him too. You're both wondering what it could be and decide to look thoroughly into the problem. Your neighbor suspects that the people next door have been remodeling their house and many people were in and out of the roads. You go in and talk to them and find out that the lumber truck was delivering building materials and when going around the corner accidentally spilled some lumber and a box of nails fell down, burst open and scattered all over the road. They thought they had picked them all up but some were left unnoticed. You clean it all up and no more flat tire for you or your neighbor. Your problem was cured because you removed the nails (cause).

This is how it works with anything and everything including your health. We have to get to the real cause because the cure is in it. Nature's law of cause and effect works constantly regardless of luck, fate, race, color, money, etc. This is a fact not a man made scam, dogma or bureaucratic rule. Nature is just. Nothing just happens. Happening is just.

This is why there are no diseases without a cause and that includes so called incurable diseases too. When you stumble on any problem (nails) in your life remember what caused it will also cure it by removing it. It is not luck, it is awareness.

We had a neighbor who was retired from the movie industry full of stories from Hollywood of fortunes and misfortunes. He personally knew many movie stars: Marilyn Monroe, Clark Gable, James Dean, etc. They all had their life stories and I loved listening to him on our daily walks. One day he was telling me that his doctor wanted him to have a quadruple by-pass surgery as soon as he recuperated from having a kidney removed. The doctor promised him that if he had the surgery he would be like a new man and could live another sixty-five years. If I didn't know any better and in my early twenties, I would have said what about two for the price of one. I tried very hard to talk him out of it but he loved parties and the good life and he wanted to be around for another sixty-five years. He knew the risk of surgery but he did not know that if he didn't change his smoking, drinking and over-eating habits that his surgery wouldn't help at all, in fact it would make things worse in a very short time. I remember asking him when he had his kidney removed to change his diet but he truly believed his doctor that his diet had nothing to do with it.

It appeared that the "nail" on the road was not the cause of his problem. This man was not aware. He decided to have the quadruple by-pass surgery anyway. When I went to visit him in the hospital he was in grave condition and he barely lived through it. He was in constant pain and could not walk with me again. He was very stressed and started to drink and smoke again and eat the same foods that caused his problem. A few months later he died. I miss him and remember his Hollywood stories. There are many others that do the same thing without looking to the cause.

Take a look at the real cause of the common cold. We do not understand it because we have to realize that each cold is the body's end – point of tolerance for toxic acids and debris. When we stop creating toxic material in the body, we will stop manifestation of the common cold. You did not catch it from your friend, co-worker or neighbor, your earned it when your body got plugged up with debris and eventually had to get rid of it and it surfaced in the form of a cold. Once you become conscious of the problem (question) your Nature directs you in what to do and what steps to take. The only time this does not occur is if we are confused or have the wrong question in mind. The problem in life is not in receiving answers but being unable to identify the right question. Once you get the question right, the answer always comes. Solutions become inevitable. The cure surfaces because you are aware of the cause (problem).

Internal hygiene, all possible improvements of heredity and lifestyle are the keynote to the health of future generations. When a young person is having serious health problems now, what can we expect of that person's offspring one or two generations ahead? This is of most concern to me. I see it every day working with young innocent children that did not have a true information and guidance toward a natural path.

Cause and effect: the body's reactions to what we do to it
How to get to the heart of the problem

Remember, whenever you have any health problem, in order to correct it, **you must look to the cause**. The cure is in the cause. Likely, one or all of these reasons are key:

1) Prescription drugs and medications are one of the problems. Besides eating genetically engineered, lifeless (dead), chemically tainted, processed foods that don't supply the elements, nutrients, energy, enzymes and vitamins you need to keep organs functioning at optimum levels;

2) You're unable to take up the nutrients a particular organ needs, due to lack of enzymes, an overworked pancreas, poor absorption and poor assimilation;

3) You're unable to eliminate toxic waste properly due to poor circulation and poor nutrition (not enough fiber and moisture). This plugs the body, impacting toxic waste and debris which is helping the parasites to thrive and that affects you physically and mentally;

4) Your brain has to have the proper nutrients to think clearly. In other words the pituitary has to orchestrate the other glands so that the whole system can function in harmony.

Fixing all this is easy by becoming aware and educating yourself. You don't really need anyone's help, especially from those who don't believe we are what we eat and what we can absorb. In other words - most doctors. Simply stop doing what made you this way, and follow Nature's wisdom. Wild animals don't have degenerative diseases because they eat what Nature intended for them: fresh, organic in its original, non-processed food form. Period. You can, too. You can be healthy without surgery, drugs, quick fixes, or depression. You can reverse almost any degenerative disease - if not completely, at least to the point it won't get any worse, only better. Let's see what we need, why, and how it all reverts to the cause.

Example one:
For eye problems and better vision

Carrots and also all yellow, orange and red fruits and vegetables contain beta-carotene. Not just for the eyes, but to prevent heart attacks, strokes, and aid many other organs, cells and capillaries. Beta-carotene nourishes the eye's blood vessels and helps with circulation, fighting the formation of cataracts.

Dark green, leafy vegetables like spinach, chard, kale, broccoli, cabbage, lettuce, etc. These contain high levels of lutein-carotenoids that help form the yellow center of the retina, the macula, responsible for slowing the progress of macular degeneration.

Garlic increases the level of selenium, a key anti-oxidant. It also keeps viral and bacterial infections under control, and is an excellent immune booster. A few cloves of fresh garlic chopped into your salad dressing every day will not only "keep the evil spirits away", but your immune system strong so you won't contract eye infections like conjunctivitis, sties, other ocular weaknesses and benefits to the whole body.

Fats are necessary for many bodily functions. Olives, avocados, seeds, nuts, and flax seed oil are good sources of the proper fat needed. Make sure the oils are organic, cold-pressed and fresh. They become rancid quickly, so keep them refrigerated. Omega-3 oils are crucial for sharp vision. They regulate eye pressure, constriction of blood vessels, blood thinning, moistening of the eye, as well as relieving eyestrain and reducing sun sensitivity. They also protect your heart, among many other functions.

Fresh fruits like blueberries are excellent for the eyes. They improve night vision by strengthening the rhodopsin, or visual purple, that keeps your vision sharper at night, and reduces glare. Blueberries are good for memory and blood as well. Other dark blue and purple fruits are good for the eyes and the whole body. Eat all you want, especially when they're in season and organic. The important thing to remember is that food eaten in its original form can be absorbed easier with all its vital elements intact for easier digestion and assimilation.

For eyes, and other organs, many doctors recommend concentrated forms and doses of natural nutrients that also help when the body can't absorb properly and has been nutritionally depleted for a long period of time. Fresh is still best - your body needs fresh food to be kept pure and free of accumulated toxic debris so extra mucus doesn't form and plug the capillaries.

Please avoid over-the-counter, commercial eye drops. They "take the red out" by shrinking blood vessels and also dilate the pupils. In addition, they have been linked to a certain form of glaucoma, known as "lack of angle closure" glaucoma. The drops have a rebound effect and wear off, leaving eyes again dry and red. After a while the eyes don't respond any longer to the drops, but damage continues. Don't treat the symptom, treat the cause. Like inhalers, and nasal sprays, eye drops don't work for long, and you must increase the dosage over time to gain the original effect. Think of the side effects and the cause first.

Allergy drugs, medications, improper food, lack of good fats, soft drinks, alcohol, and coffee (diuretics) pull fluids out of your body. They dehydrate the body and mucus lining, and make your eyes itchy, dry, red, and burning. Symptom-treating medications are the biggest culprit. Some homeopathic medicines are excellent in treating conjunctivitis, and for burning, itching eyes (Apis). You can find them in health food stores.

For painful and light-sensitive eyes, you can use Belladonna. For allergies and discharge, as well as eyes that are "glued" shut you can use Euphrasia. Vitamin A drops are excellent for conjunctivitis. If you have twitching in your eyes, or other places on your face or body, try 400 mg of magnesium. Twitching is a simple sign you're low on the magnesium that nourishes nerves and muscles. Be sure to get magnesium glycine for best absorption.

A variety of fresh fruits and vegetables remain the best form of prevention and cure.

You won't need glasses if your body is in perfect health, plus there are simple exercises that will strengthen eye muscles. With head straight, move eyes side to side three times; up and down three times; and diagonally three times. Avoid any strain while doing this exercise. Do it slowly, and gradually. Improvements will be amazing. I've never worn glasses, and never will. My grandmother didn't, even at the age of ninety-three.

There is a story later in the book about a man who improved his vision sixty-five percent! He improved his eating habits and cleansed his body so well that in two to three months his absorption became more efficient. His eyes finally received more of what they needed and his vision improved sixty-five percent. His doctor called it a miracle. I believe even **miracles** have a cause. Don't let anyone fool you. There aren't any quick fixes and magic pills. However, consider three months great progress.

Example two:
For sinus problems (sinusitis)

Millions suffer to no avail, unaided in the long-term by surgery or medications. Yet the solution is simple if you look to the cause. Eat right and avoid mucus-forming foods like milk, butter, cheese, pastries, other sugar-filled sweets, as well as genetically engineered foods that are messing up our core (DNA). What other consequences can we expect in the future? Red meat, in addition to being laden with hormones and chemicals, is hard to get through the digestive tract where it causes bowel pockets and putrefaction. Fried foods are loaded with TFA (trans-fatty acids), which are very clogging and dangerous and will be mentioned later. TFA leaks out all through the intestines and penetrates every organ causing havoc in the form of allergies, and hardening of the capillary walls. Beer isn't the best thing for sinuses either. It contains molds that aggravate sinus problems.

For sinus support, you can add garlic, onions, cayenne pepper, mustard, and horseradish with lemon - to expel mucus, pineapple enzyme, papaya juice, herb tea, and olive leaf extract. Try rinsing out your nose with real seawater. But before you try any of these, start putting good fresh stuff in and keep your system clean and pure. Look to the possible cause.

You're going to say: What's left? The fun is gone. Variety is the key - fresh fruits and vegetables, seeds, nuts, and herbs. Does that really sound like *nothing* is left? Don't overlook the beautiful rainbow color and incredible taste, shape, and form Nature provides. Check the recipes in Chapter Six for ideas. Besides are we only here living to eat or are we eating to live obsessed with devitalized food yet starved?

You can join my "uncooking crusade" and learn how to have fun with good produce while discovering how excellent it tastes. Email me at: DRRUZA@hotmail.com

Please understand this: it doesn't matter if the problem is with the eyes, sinuses, prostate, or immune system . . . it's all *one* body. What needs to be healed will heal. Nature knows what to do, and how to balance your body. What caused it will heal it by removing the problem. However, when you put the brakes on by confusing the body with chemicals, pesticides, steroids, hormones, and processed lifeless foods, the body plugs up and produces toxicity in your system. It does not allow the body to heal naturally.

True, different nutrients, elements, and vitamins are needed for different organs and their optimal functioning. The thyroid needs iodine. The brain needs B vitamins. The prostate needs zinc. **The point is**, when you eat a variety of whole foods, they have some, and often all, of the essential elements you're made of. Different colored fruits and vegetables have the vibrational energy that heals the whole body, corresponds with innate intelligence in your pituitary gland and hypothalamus that orchestrates the whole body. How can you do it if it's out of balance and doesn't know which signal to respond to?

The health of the body is only as good as the health, collectively, of **all the body's individual cells**. In turn, the health of the cells is determined by the quality of the lymph fluids that bathe the cells, which is in turn dependent on the purity of the bloodstream. So dirty blood, or toxemia, is the culprit. The DNA and RNA cannot produce healthy cells.

The composition of the blood is complex and is maintained by the combined action of all the vital organs. The liver redistributes digested foods into the bloodstream to help with the rest of the body's requirements. The liver and kidneys receive, via blood, the waste products of all cells, and throw it out in the urinary and other elimination organs. For the maintenance of correct blood sugar levels, the liver depends on information from the pancreas, which not only secretes insulin and glycogen used in the control of blood sugar, but **also secretes** the primary **digestive enzyme juices** used in the vital digestion of the foods we eat.

Like it or not, the main status of your health is determined entirely by the foods you eat. It will even effect your thoughts and emotions. Food is key to your health. No one can decide for you what you eat. The body will respond accordingly. Consequences! Think about it. Food is the foundation of good health. Your life is a manifestation of the food you eat. Call it a miracle if you will.

We need to learn what good food is. We need to teach our doctors that processed food has *everything* to do with disease and symptoms.

The natural digestive process utilizes enzymes that exist in raw organic foods which, when food is eaten, performs a considerable amount of pre-digestion (food is broken down with saliva) before the main digestive system in the stomach gets to work on it. This means a huge workload is taken off the pancreas -the organ that produces the main supply of digestive juices and enzymes.

You can clearly see this natural benefit is missing when cooked food is consumed. Cooking *destroys* enzymes, double-penalizing the pancreas, making it work harder and become more enlarged compared to when you eat raw food. Imagine what happens when you deep-fry your food and eat meat three times a day. Pancreatic cancer is rising incredibly faster than any other. You can clearly see why. Many people have diabetes and don't even realize it.

The best recovery from chronic, incurable diseases is made on diets composed of raw organic fruits and vegetables. Living foods are medicines - life sources that are in constant connection with the universal intelligence - God. When vital organs are at their lowest stage of function (easy digestion), only such a diet makes it possible for the organ to provide proper body chemistry and maintain health. Clearly, raw food provides the maximum benefit to both the sick and healthy harmonizing the body and spirit.

Being a vegetarian isn't enough. You must become an eater of more raw food. Eating raw provides the least wear and tear, and the least "silting up" of body organs and tissues. Fruits remain the best and easiest of foods to digest.

Old age and disease can be deferred by selecting food that provides the least amount of harmful residue, by eating smaller quantities. Through moderation in lifestyle habits the body will continue to heal itself.

The quality of the cellular environment is the determining factor in how healthy and how long a person will live. If you want to feel a bit better, eliminate the most harmful substances from your diet. If you want to be exceptionally healthy, enlightened, and live a long time - eat to live, instead of live to eat. Less is more. Put the highest quality organic fruits and vegetables, sprouted grains, seeds and nuts (that are soaked first) in your body. This is what you need to thrive. It will also help you to think more clearly, positively and harmoniously in tune with universal intelligence. **Cause and cure are one.** The choice is yours.

It will be very beneficial to transition slowly to a fifty-fifty raw-cooked diet and slowly move to seventy-thirty by getting gradually accustomed to eighty-twenty and further if desired.

Excuses are always found until you realize that you're in charge and you cannot blame anyone anymore, not even your doctor because most have no clue about nutrition.

Education by example is the best way. Living our teaching. Making our lives our message. Healing takes place while a person is well. After an illness has set in, it is much harder. When it comes to preventing or reversing disease lack of enzymes are our worst enemy. Many people are totally unaware that enzymes are found only in raw food. Enzymes enable your body to break down the vitamins, minerals, proteins, carbohydrates, fats and hormones into the substances your body needs to function, grow and rejuvenate. When your body has to compensate by working harder and harder, disease sets in.

Humans Are Engineered Raw
(With permission from: *Nature's First Law*, by Arlin, Dini and Wolfe)

"To live simply and naturally is the highest and final goal."
Friedrich Nietzsche

There can be only three reasons why a machine would break down: incidental wear and tear coming in from the outside, a flaw exists in its design, and/or a deficiency exists in the raw materials required to run the machine.

Incidental damage sustained by the human organism from external sources (burns, injuries, poisoning, etc.) is easily understood and there is no disagreement on the holistic methods to be employed in their treatments. These external damages may include all needle-administered drugs, vitamin pills, mineral supplements, alcohol, THC, tainted water, as well as those innumerable poisons introduced into the body by eating or breathing in cooked, dead, and denatured substances.

Every organism's design pattern is found in its DNA code. The genetic blueprint for the human organism has been damaged by countless millennia of unnatural feeding. The DNA code continues to be assaulted at an ever-increasing pace. DNA damage is passed down from generation to generation and the flaws accumulate. With bad breeding they make their outward appearance. Genetic damage is a one-way path into an abyss from which there is no return.

The most harmonious raw materials for the human organism are the raw plant food created by Nature. Even the slightest alteration in the type of food designed for the organism means dislocating the proper operations of the human organism - it means disease. This is an unerring axiom of Nature.

Living forces have constructed the raw materials intended for the human machine with such precise calculations that when a raspberry is placed in the mouth, it breaks up and spreads throughout the organism, fulfilling all its needs. That berry first builds the rudimentary structures of the simple cells. It then constructs all the internal machinery and mechanisms of the differentiated cells. That raspberry provides the materials necessary for cleaning and lubricating all the component parts of the organism. It renews damaged cells, replaces old and tired cells with youthful organelles. It warms the body, supplies fuel for the organism, and any other task demanded of it. Just as every design engineer specifies, through detailed calculations, the raw materials necessary for a machine, so has Nature specified the requisite raw materials essential for humans and all other living creatures.

Because the human organism has an extremely intricate construction, its raw materials are of a correspondingly complex design, consisting of a myriad of organic molecules.

By its unfailing wisdom, Nature has combined within the structures of living fruits, vegetables, and herbs all those raw materials required by the human organism. Each of those materials has its precise quantity. Thus, of one kind of substance, we may need a gram, of another, a thousandth of a gram. This is the operative rule for all organisms. It is essential that those materials should always be at the disposal of the cells in their predetermined ratios and quantities. Special care must be taken to insure that none of them is absent from the aggregate whole.

It is interesting to note that all living creatures, from a termite to a shark, from a mountain lion to a giraffe, recognize their natural foods and make full use of them to satisfy their nutritional needs. Paradoxically enough, humans are the only creatures to abandon their instincts and completely lose sight of those indispensable foods essential for their well being. Cooked food has completely divorced humanity from its instincts.

People labor day and night in laboratories and research institutes. They conduct all kinds of useless tests and experiments to discover "natural" materials. They then manufacture them by processing raw plant foods, dead animals, or by synthesizing them artificially. Strange names are concocted for these substances. Huge multilevel-marketing companies are then formed to distribute these products all over the world, so people can be "nourished." And this is called "all-natural."

A breakfast cereal company that labels a product "100% Natural" is lying through its cooked teeth. What is natural about

cooked grain? How about "0% Natural?"
     Without realizing what they are doing, scientists have come into direct conflict with Nature. Blinded by addictions, these researchers are unable to see that Nature has compiled the highest forms of nutrients within countless types of fruits and vegetables. Nature has spread these all over the world, especially in the tropical zones where Homo sapiens originated.
     Cooked food is poison.

I often see young children that are depleted of enzymes and can no longer digest their food properly due to lack of raw food. Our liver and pancreas are designed to store enzymes if needed in case of emergency, but today that storage is depleted and the pancreas has to work much harder. This is why so many young people have health problems and allergies so early in life. Juvenile diabetes among other degenerative diseases is becoming rampant.

Lack of enzymes puts stress on all vital organs. When your body works so much harder at making up for the missing nutrients it short changes all of your internal systems. Arthritis, high blood pressure, obesity and chronic fatigue are just a few of the health problems related to this deficiency. Just zinc triggers over two hundred enzymes for growth, immunity and sexual development. Selenium works with enzymes for protein metabolism and healthy hormonal balance. Chromium helps support healthy blood sugar levels and manganese aids enzymes to break down and use carbohydrates.

Our body is not just one thing, it is a combination of many things. People need to realize that when you eat a whole apple that apple has perfect balance of all elements, vitamins and nutrients even protein. How can that apple not do the body good? But when you eat an apple pie with ice cream on top your body has to process all that combination of stuff and isolate the things it cannot use. It then stores it causing burden on the whole system so in order to keep the system alkaline it has to pull the calcium out of the bones in order to compensate for the sugar in the pie and the ice cream.

All Raw Plants Are Complete Foods
(with permission from: *Nature's First Law*,
by Arlin, Dini, Wolfe)

"The whole is more than the sum of its parts."

Goethe

Every mammal must eat raw plant food - especially green leaves. All mammalian carnivores are really omnivores. Dogs must eat grass, and not just when they are ill, as popular myth dictates. Cats dig up and chew on plant roots. Brown bears typically eat 95% plant food. The reason for this is that all raw plant foods are whole. They completely nourish the body. All food chains begin with plant forms. It makes no difference what raw plant foods a species has an affinity for. What is important is that the food consumed is living, natural, and intact.

When a thoroughbred horse feeds on grass, nobody ever worries the animal may suffer from an insufficiency of proteins or minerals. Animals too, like humans, need every kind of vitamin, mineral, enzyme, etc. which arise from the life-giving soil. How is it that a moose can grow into a fantastic creature on simple grass, and that a human cannot do the same on raw fruits and vegetables?

Everybody can clearly see the food choices made by the myriad of animals populating the Earth consist of a limited variation. They are designed to get the foods they enjoy most and that are in their immediate vicinity. Nevertheless, we are not able to find even a single case of avitaminosis or any other nutritional deficiency among them.

If you take the foodstuffs consumed by those animals into the laboratories of biologists, in each of them they will find several substances of varying qualities and quantities. They will then tell you that in a particular plant there is so much protein, so much fat, and so much of one vitamin or another. Thus in each plant they will enumerate some arbitrary number of constituents they have managed to find and will carefully determine their quantities one by one. Even in the richest fruits the number of constituents they have succeeded in discovering has been strictly limited. In reality, this does not prove that each of those foodstuffs consists of only the dozen or so constituents they have found; rather, it is an indication that their technical skills and resources are quite inadequate to fully analyze and to determine qualitatively and quantitatively all those constituents that have come together in Nature's laboratory. It means that in a particular food they have been able to discover only those few kinds of constituents; the rest have remained hidden from them.

The main reason for this is the fact that the substances discovered by biologists are not the primary constituents of those plant bodies, but they are compounds appearing in different form in different plant bodies. Upon entering the animal body, those compounds are broken down to the molecular level and synthesized again. Thus, new compounds are formed corresponding to the needs of the organism.

All plant forms consumed by animals consist of the same basic constituents. Fundamentally, all plants consist of three main classes of substances.

The first of them is living water, which is familiar to us all. One cannot live without water. We may well remember that the purest and safest source of water is found in plant bodies - especially fruit. Plant water has been vivified and electrified by sunlight. Humans, like all the other primates, need very little water because their food has such a high-water content. In Nature, we see mountain gorillas drinking by dipping a hand into a running stream and sucking the water off the hairs on the back of their hand. Due to the massive pollution of nearly all water sources on the planet, one should only drink collected rain water, eat snow, or distilled water (an unnatural creation, but useful in extreme circumstances) if fruit or plant juice is not obtainable. Never drink bottled spring waters in the United States because, by law, they need only be 50% spring water, the rest can be ordinary tap water. People drink exorbitant amounts of water to dilute the dehydrated, cooked-food extracts that fill their bodies. There really is no need to ever drink a glass of water as long as you are 100% raw and eat mostly high-water-content fruits and vegetables. Nature's reaction to internal pollution is to dilute toxic materials with water.

The second class consists of fiber, or roughage. This substance, cellulose, constitutes the framework of plants, giving them form and firmness. Fiber is not completely broken down and assimilated in the animal organism; it is typically expelled from the body in the form of feces. It is, however, an essential part of the animal diet. If there were no roughage in the food consumed by animals, their intestines would have nothing to expel, and in the course of time they would shrivel and dry up. Yet, many people are so shortsighted that, regarding fiber as "indigestible," they deliberately remove it from their foodstuffs, as a result of which nearly all humankind suffers from constipation. The causes of constipation are the absence of roughage in the diet and cooked-food clogging.

The last of the three classes of plant substances is the nutrient itself - the juice - which is fully digestible and can be completely assimilated by the animal organism.

The essential differences between diverse plant bodies arise from variations in the relative quantities of those three classes of substances. Thus, the main difference between the common grass and fruit is that in grass, fiber and chlorophyll predominate, whereas fruit consists of only a moderate amount of roughage, with plenty of concentrated nutriments and an adequate supply of living water. Because of the special structure of their digestive organs and their faculty of rumination, grazing herbivores are able to crush and grind the grass, to extract the nutrients dispersed in it and to expel the rest from their bodies. This is how certain animals manage to obtain nourishment from dry hay or straw; the camel is able to sustain life on desert thistles and the donkey on the roughest of grasses.

From this we can draw the important conclusion that all plant forms contain the necessary nutrients for sustaining animal organisms. In some plants they appear in a scattered form, in others they are highly concentrated. Among natural foods the most nutritious are avocados, bananas, cherimoya, grapes, lemons, mangos, nectarines, oranges, peaches, strawberries, tomatoes, watermelons, and all the other seeded fruits. After which come the herbs and greens.

Those nutritive constituents found in a concentrated state in the fruit of a tree are also found dispersed sparsely in leaves, bark, and branches. A giant animal like the giraffe nourishes itself by feeding on tree leaves. When a small bud of a tree is grafted upon another tree, it shoots forth branches and eventually gives the corresponding fruit. This is a clear indication that a bud contains all the elementary constituents essential for the formation of a given fruit.

Now what are those elementary constituents? They are the atoms, which may be regarded as the smallest chemically indivisible particle of an element that can take part in a chemical change, and the molecules, which are the smallest particles of a compound. All edible plants consist of almost the same elements arranged in different proportions to form various compounds. They only differ from one another in form, color, and taste. Thus, clover and sheep are exactly the same. On being introduced into the stomach of a sheep, the molecular structure of clover undergoes a metamorphosis and becomes the sheep. There is a similar correspondence between fruit and humans.

All plant and animal life is nothing but an eternal interchange and circulation of atoms. It is here that the infinite wisdom of Nature asserts itself. We throw onto the ground a tiny seed. After a few days it sprouts. Then it shoots forth branches and leaves. In due course it gives fruit. Later that fruit is changed into an ant, a wild sow, or a human that roams about this world for a while and then returns its atoms to the Earth. There, under the vivifying influence of sunlight, those very atoms are revived afresh, new life is breathed into them and they are turned once more into the same plants and animals, to repeat the everlasting cycle of life over and over again. This cycle of life is severely altered by the toxic nature of dead, decomposing, cooked-food humans. They are literally "pushing down the daisies."

The same principles of nutrition that hold true for animals also hold true for plants. Plants get diseases when there are no longer any elements in the soil to supply them with their nutritional demands. Plants also become subject to diseases when toxins, poisons, and artificial chemicals leach into their root or respiratory structures, filter into their living fluids, and become trapped in their plant fibers.

In order that plant food may give birth to specialized, healthy, and highly-evolved cells, it must not only be complete and living but it must also be active. For example, wheatberries should be sprouted (activated) before consumption. It must be said that humans are not a "sproutarian" species. Sprouts cannot sustain you in the long-term, but raw fruits and green-leafed vegetables can. Sprouts are recognized here as the plant growth stage before leaves are formed; once leaves are formed on the sprout we consider it a green-leafed vegetable. Sprouts have an affinity for water. When they are ingested, they dehydrate the digestive organs of the body. They may clog the body's waste elimination system much like cooked food. Sprout consumption should be limited to the winter season.

Experience has shown us house birds are not satisfied with dry seeds alone. They demand some fresh food as well. The particular variety of those seeds or the fresh food is not important. Perfect nourishment can be obtained by choosing a certain variety of seed or grain and supplementing it with any fresh fruit or soft vegetable.

This fact brings us to the important conclusion that the most perfect food ceases to be perfect after it is dried. Keeping this in mind, it is truly mind-boggling that people regard those substances that come out of ovens, microwaves, toasters, boxes, cans, boiling water, and the jaws of roaring machines as nourishment.

Nevertheless, animal organisms (including natural humans) do not suffer serious harm when they are deprived of fresh foods during the few months of winter. For they make up the deficiency during the bountiful spring and summer, when all Nature comes to life again. Nature has insured them to that mode of life.

Nuts and seeds are indeed living foodstuffs. Many are palatable and edible in their natural, raw state, such as macadamias, almonds, and sunflower seeds. Others can easily be aroused, activated, and turned into perfect foods by being soaked in water...

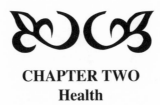

CHAPTER TWO
Health

"The preservation of health is a duty. Few seem conscious that there is such a thing as physical morality."
Herbert Spencer

Health is wealth. As in other branches of life itself, truly without it there is little left.

Some say that digestion is the greatest secret of life. Some say that the mind is the key to health. Some say that cheerfulness is the best promoter of health. I agree with all of these in a sense, but in order to have healthy mind, you have to have a healthy body. In order to have a healthy body, you have to ingest the proper nutrients in their organic state, so that body can use what it needs and when, this way the mind can orchestrate the body. Without biology there is no psychology.

Health means harmony, happiness, success, love, and liberty. All in one truth. All in all.

"Oh, health! Health is the blessing of the rich! The riches of the poor! Who can sit by thee at too dear a rate, since there is no enjoying this world without thee?"
Ben Johnson

For some reason I was fascinated with health from the earliest time I can recall - perhaps four years old. We did not have doctors where I lived and my family made sure we never needed one. I do not remember even getting sick as a child. We lived with Nature and in harmony with the seasons. Health meant life, a normal state of being. My first realization of health and life became unavoidable when I asked my father where my grandfathers were, and why I'd never seen them. My father explained they died in the war before I was born. Of course I wanted to know everything. If I would ever see them, how their deaths happened, etc.

I became allergic to the word war. I asked my father if everyone dies, and if he and Mama would one day, too. Remembering clearly his face as if it was just a few minutes ago. He did not want to disappoint a four-year-old and politely tried to wriggle out of answering, but my persistence demanded an answer. After all, no one ever wants a father or mother to die. Some never have the chance to meet their grandfathers. Now I know why I cried when my son was born. I did not want him to have to go to war.

I sat in my father's lap, looked him straight in the eye and asked him again: "Papa, are you going to die some day?" He answered: "Well ... a long time from now, but by the time you grow up people will find out that the cure for all disease is in the cause, and you will never have to die of disease."

Right there and then I wanted to hurry and grow up so I could find the cause. That way if my Papa ever got sick he wouldn't have to die either!

My father was well known for telling the truth. He was my idol and I believed him. He would never lie to me and if he did not know something, he would find out. For me it was enough to know that there was a cure for all disease and that people did not have to die of disease. The cure was always there; people just did not know it! The **Cure** was and always will be in the **Cause**. There could also be more than one cause. I have a hard time getting this fact across to most people. Yet it is so simple and you will find out why that is.

Well, now I know it. My father was right. With every fiber of my being I believe that the cure for all disease lies in Nature's law of cause and effect. There is no such thing as an incurable disease. People die of disease because of their addiction to improper diet, drugs (both legal and illegal), wrong, stressful lifestyle and a combination of many complex causes.

Can you imagine if every child was told what my father told me? That there is a cure for every disease. Proof is what you need now, and I'm more than ready to give it to you. Hopefully you are starting to realize it and things are starting to make more sense.

One reason why our health today is such an immense mess is

because people are not able to think straight. This is due to the fact we put the false messages in our brains and depleted, processed foods in our bodies. When Albert Schwitzer, two times a Nobel Prize winner, was asked what was wrong with man today, his simple answer was: "Man simply doesn't think." I agree totally, but I want to know why. When we analyze why it will go back to the roots of improper nutrition, and the incorrect input or false information we constantly feed ourselves - to the point we become confused, physically and mentally. The brain is not giving correct chemical signals to the glands that produce the proper hormonal balance so the body may function harmoniously. How can we put the wrong fuel in an engine and expect it to perform well?

Indeed, the preservation of health is our duty to ourselves and our children, the innocent ones. Only a few of us seem conscious there is such a thing as physical morality and what we ingest, and even fewer, that they are connected as one in our daily lives. Cure and cause are one. Morally we owe the truth to our future generations so that they don't make the same mistakes we have.

"The bend in the road is not the end of the road."
Dr. Bernard Jensen

Does health mean disease-free? Yes, yet so many are unhealthy. In fact, there are very few people who *are* healthy, but are rather "getting by" with prescription drugs, surgery, hormones and quick fixes and most don't know how healthy really feels.

"Health" is a big business that has turned into the even bigger business of disease care, all due to the poor eating habits and prescription drugs that treat symptoms but not cause. This combined with poor nutrition and absorption of nutrients along with eating devitalized food further contributes to disease.

Many organizations such as chemical, unnatural big vitamin manufacturers, drug companies, publications and health newsletters, to mention but a few, are literally thriving on so-called new preventions. What good is achieved by searching, wasting precious time and money, and purposely ignoring the real cause? A simple truth.

Health is a simple truth. You are what you eat and what you absorb, and what comes out of you, that is, if you are not constipated!

Ask yourself once and for all why you have aches and pains? Why you haven't felt good for so long that you've actually forgotten what good feels like? Why you really have PMS, allergies, arthritis, need a hysterectomy, etc? It is time to admit that they all come about little by little as a manifestation of your body trying to tell you something because it's deprived of simple, wholesome nutrients and loaded with toxic chemicals and metals.

Nobody in this whole wide world can prove me wrong. This is unavoidable truth. We have been fooled, misinformed and lied to due to ulterior motives.

What's nice is this can all be corrected by eating a simple diet of non-processed living foods, the way Nature made them for us, with a wide variety available everywhere. It is also helpful to eat in moderation and only when we are hungry. None of this "don't skip breakfast" stuff. In fact, breakfast means breaking your fast from not eating all night. It should be skipped or eaten lightly. The liver, which removes toxins from our blood stream, detoxifies itself from midnight to noon, and needs the break. That's why most of us aren't hungry when we get up in the morning. If you find you are hungry, eat some fresh fruit. Take advantage of your body's natural processes and your body will take care of you.

Worry does not help, so quit worrying and have a purpose in life. Help someone in need. Think good thoughts. I guarantee your troubles will go away. These troubles are all related to one another and are a chain reaction to improper daily living. Be honest. Admit it once and for all, take action and watch miracles happen!

Today we are looking for quick fixes. Let's face it, most people who are taking pills, drugs and vitamins are hoping one pill will take care of their problems, not knowing that they are actually consuming synthesized chemicals the body can't absorb. Most of the vitamins you find on the shelf even have false labeling, calling them "natural" and "organic." Get the best kind at the health food store. How can the body use and metabolize this manmade chemical stuff? It can't. Degenerative diseases are increasing rapidly. Millions more will die as they gorge on synthetic vitamins in the name of health.

Starvation from malnutrition is nothing more than constantly eating empty food calories without proper enzymes. These foods produce false energy and make us fat, but are completely devoid of the nutritional value without which we cannot survive, but rather, develop degenerative diseases. Dietary deficiencies definitely make us more susceptible to disease, general weakening of the bodily functions down to cellular degeneration.

The key to true health is fresh organic food, education and awareness not the treatment of symptoms. We are so misinformed and unaware.

"The constitution of man's body has not changed to meet the new conditions of his artificial environment that has replaced his natural one. The result is that of perpetual discord between man and his environment. The effect of this discord is general deterioration of man's body, the symptoms of which are termed disease."

Dr. Hilton Hotema

A man of thirty-five came to see me in desperation after his doctor told him he could not help him any longer. The doctor had said the young man had a very short time to live: two weeks to two months. When I asked what he was eating and drinking he replied: "My doctor told me that I have colon and liver cancer, and it has spread all over, but food has nothing to do with it. They took my bowel out and installed a radiation pump in my liver to reduce the tumors. Statistically my doctor said I am history. I am desperate now. My kids need me. Can you please help me?" I answered yes, if he would allow me to teach him that he did not have to die and that what he ate and drank along with his stress and his thoughts had everything to do with the disease he had including being a criminal attorney, the most stressful job I've heard off.

He became a believer. Eighteen months later he called and told me he had to go back to work. His unemployment had expired due to the fact he no longer had cancer! He didn't feel like going back to his law firm. He hated lying for people and didn't want that kind of stress any longer. I suggested he seek his real purpose in life and find something he loved. He didn't know what that could be. I said: help someone like you. Thousands are dying unaware there is a possible cure for their disease.

Can you imagine a doctor telling his patient he statistically has two months to live and that diet had nothing to do with the man's grave condition? This is why a doctor has to go to school for so long - long enough to get completely brainwashed into having no sense at all. Into believing that nutrition has nothing to do with our state of health. Can you believe this kind of nonsense?

In reality, this is what I hear when I ask people about their problem. Ninety-five percent are told by their doctors food has nothing to do with their problems. I am shocked. Why do people even bother to eat then? And what is it that people eat and think that causes them to get cancer?

It certainly seems that the majority of people eat cooked and processed food that has no healing power at all. So when a doctor says that the food has nothing to do with their disease, it means that the dead food has no healing power. It still has everything to do with their condition but if they want to get better eating non-processed organic food will have everything to do with whether they live or die. In other words the difference is not just food and diet but the fact that it has to be living food - not dead food (devitalized).

Health is being taught in few places today. Other than a few universities and some private colleges that teach mandatory classes on the subject, there are no courses in *true* nutrition. Check www. treeoflife.com for true nutrition classes.

Disease is handled by treating the symptoms. Modern medicine treats symptoms only, not the cause. How can we possibly get better? If we did, of course, doctors would close their surgical and prescription practices. This is the reason they use statistics to cloud the truth. If you do not pay attention to your diet, you will become a statistic too. The irony is that most doctors do not even know this. They are unaware.

There are many other so-called natural therapies and varying branches of treatments for different diseases which we will discuss in depth later. But if these too only treat symptoms, we are wasting precious time again. We are simply beating around the bush. How can that be, you might ask yourself? The kindest answer I can give you is not just money or greed, but sadly, complete unawareness, an inability to think clearly because of the constant bombardment of lies we are taught in school and at home. Along with lack of alive, raw, organic nutrients in their own diet is what causes the brain not to make sense so ignorance sets in.

Naturopathy and nutrition are but two treatments that can get to the real root of a problem other than corrective surgery or accidents.

I am not saying that other natural therapies aren't good, many can help as you will see. But the key here is that all the others will not completely get to the bottom of the problem if they do not include the cause - organic nutrition.

It boggles the mind that a doctor can pass his medical exam without ever taking nutritional class. He is never even exposed to the principle cause of disease and the simple truth. Doctors need to become more aware. They need to study health and nutrition, then there would be fewer diseases left to study.

Doctors are unaware genetic disorders are due not only to inherited tendencies but by the habits we are bequeathed as well, including poor nutrition. We literally are heir to our parents' suicidal addictions.

I know and believe we can improve and strengthen any inherited weakness within the body by supporting weak organs with proper nutrition, good organic raw fruits, vegetables and herbs. If we do not take nutrition into account, but fall back on drugs and surgery, our inherited weaknesses will kill us. The new generation will have even bigger problems. Those problems will show up in younger offspring, sooner than it did in previous generations. Today, doctors are telling eighteen year-olds that it's normal to remove their gall bladder, uterus and appendix. This is the truth I hear from innocent people who come to see me out of desperation. Their health insurance does not cover a visit to a naturopathic doctor or alternative therapies, the one that could help cure their problem. People have been continuing to miss the key that opens the right door to our health and happiness.

Because of this simple and yet total unawareness of the truth, many new theories, techniques and quick fixes have emerged to "help" us with our disease, constant pain and suffering. All this is to no avail until we look the problem straight in the eye. Without finding the cause, people will continue to suffer. Having one more surgery will sooner or later lead to another and yet another. Why? Because you did not look to the cause of your first surgery and you did not put live food in your body so the mind is confused in orchestrating the body.

In fact things are getting so bad I was morally forced into doing something about this issue. I wrote this book knowing if this knowledge were to be kept inside of me and shared only with people that come to see me when everything else fails, the results would be lost health, lives, and unnecessary suffering.

There is a light in sight. The Journal of the American Medical Association (JAMA) says "Not only is the public dissatisfied with conventional medicine, these help-care alternatives mirrored their own values ... toward health and life." US News and World Report says " Medical schools across the US are struggling to add courses about alternative medicine ... including elite institutions like Harvard and Johns Hopkins University ... " The Journal of Family Practice reports " ... forty-seven percent of the doctors reported using alternative therapies themselves." US News and World Reports recently says that "The cure for cancer is still years away." Though America invested twenty-nine billion dollars in research, five hundred fifty-five thousand will die of cancer this year. That is ten thousand five-hundred seventy-six every week – two hundred fifteen thousand more than in 1971. Lung cancer in the last eighteen years shot up forty-two percent, breast cancer increased a hundred percent from two decades ago. Testicular cancer is up five hundred percent and most doctors are still treating and masking the symptoms as well as ignoring the real cause. I guess science has to prove whereas

Nature just is. Senseless delays can cost you your health – your life. **Please** reflect on this and stay on Nature's path.

Most of the proceeds from the sale of this book will go to kindergarten classrooms, some in the form of free books about the food we eat and what it does to us. Little children will have a true start from the beginning. This project has already begun, and you are helping by buying this book. Awareness is the key that opens the doors to health and harmony and the holistic way of life.

We have a long way to go. When I was in New Zealand recently, I was shocked to find American fast-food restaurants popping up everywhere. Worse are the advertisements claiming to help children with cancer, brain tumors, leukemia, etc. Yes, a certain amount of what these corporations earn will go to help the little ones, but what irony. The very same food kids eat at one of these places is killing them. And remember the thirty-five year-old man with liver cancer who came to see me? His diet consisted mainly of fast foods. He admitted to me that he rarely ate any fresh fruits or vegetables though his grandmother had warned him he should.

Please, whatever you think now about this information, look into it more deeply. I am not making any of this up. You don't have to be a fanatic or deprive yourself. It's okay to have junk food once in a great while, but the less you stray away from Nature, the less you will feel the need to. That I promise! Junk food is addictive. Besides ask your fast food restaurant to carry raw salads, juices and fruits so you can have at least something raw.

While we are on the subject of fast foods, I wanted to point out why they are probably the worst thing for your health and toxic to the body for several reasons. The "natural" hydrogenated oils used to make French fries are immune-depressive and highly processed with preservatives so they will not spoil or turn rancid. The process used to hydrogenate fat creates totally new molecules forced into abnormal shapes so the body does not know what to do with them. They are called trans-fatty acids, or TFA. This deformed fat is deadly stuff. The body tries to correct the deformation, and then isolates the TFA when it can't. TFA is found in all processed and fast foods. How much of this can a living body take? Every day? Two or three times a day? Give me a break! Better yet, give your body a break from fast and processed food.

As if TFA wasn't bad enough, to make food look better, manufacturers use yellow dyes. Cadmium, a toxic metal that interferes with absorption of zinc, other minerals and elements and is used in the processing of this yellow dye. So our bodies end up even hungrier for more food. "Natural" (i.e. deformed, metal-laden and toxic) hydrogenated oils are the biggest culprits of today's ill health. Are they unaware of this or is it something else in question?!

During the very high heating process, hydrogen is bubbled through the oil and forced under pressure into the boiling fat molecules in the presence of aluminum, nickel, copper, and other heavy metals. Some amounts of the metals are retained in the fat and most of the essential fatty acids (EFA) are lost. Once this is done to the oil, the oil cannot spoil any longer and a shelf life is guaranteed for infinity. When you see no expiration date, or a lengthy one, the oil has been preserved and the product has become carcinogenic. The oil will stick to your insides like glue. It makes the blood sticky (sticky blood platelets). This thick blood deposits fat including the TFA, the deformed fat, in the arteries, among other inorganic materials, in the liver, kidneys, prostate, gall bladder, and all other organs. It also makes cell membranes more permeable so other microbes can enter and destroy the cell. Also, TFA (the deformed fats) enter into the blood stream and destroy the body and arteries.

Now, we do need fat. The vast number of our approximately sixty-three trillion cells could not function without it. Fat is basic to life and builds cell membranes and nerves in our body, but when fat metabolism runs amuck, everything goes wrong. The liver uses fat to metabolize and transport many vital substances in the blood all around the body. Fat helps the blood to clot; otherwise we would bleed to death with the slightest cut. Also, hormones would not be able to be made if it wasn't for fat.

However the kind of fat we need is *monounsaturated* - not the polyunsaturated we talked about earlier. Monounsaturated is the kind of fat you find in fruits and vegetables in their original forms - non-processed. Raw cold-pressed olive oil, flax seed oil and avocados are good examples.

So it isn't fat that is killing us, like your doctor says, but the kind of fat we eat - processed and preserved like margarine, mayonnaise and those nasty hydrogenated oils.

We need essential fatty acids (EFA) because the body does not manufacture them, so we must obtain them through food like seeds, nuts, and their oils. We need EFA in order to be healthy. eighty-five percent of people do not get enough EFA. This is a major contributing factor in many disorders like allergies, attention deficit disorder (ADD), hyperactivity in children, immune system disorders, infections, wounds that won't heal, scarring, hair loss, skin problems, kidney failure, liver degeneration, atrophied glands, seizures and many other problems of today.

We need to eat real raw food like walnuts, almonds, olives, avocados, sesame seeds, flax seeds, and a variety of these kinds of EFA-rich foods.

Cholesterol is produced by the liver and is found in all body tissues and cells. Our body makes it - we must have it, we get it in our food also. Without cholesterol, we would not have hormones and our metabolism would cease to function. Cholesterol is also an antioxidant. It takes care of the problems in the blood and lubricates us where needed. The brain cannot function without cholesterol. In fact, the body will make its own if we do not take enough in with food. When we get too much, we get clogged arteries, because when we have too much inorganic calcium it mixes with the free flowing cholesterol and causes arteries and capillaries to harden.

So doctors now prescribe cholesterol-lowering drugs by the millions and recommend substituting margarine for butter. Margarine is processed oil and only leads to more trouble. The story ends sadly. Another life lost to clogged arteries that didn't need to happen.

Often doctors don't know much about nutrition or how it works. Their own average life span is fifty-six years. They recommend the same things they do for themselves. They are unfortunately unaware. Remember this. You must take matters into your own hands. Be informed and in charge of your own health.

When you are finished with this book, you will understand how simple it is to stay healthy. You will know that every cure lies in the cause, regardless of the name of the disease. When you do something wrong and continue to do wrong without realizing that you are doing it - you lose. When you know what is wrong and stop doing it, then you will win. Now you understand that **the cure is in the cause**. Can you imagine how simple this is? If you don't know what is right and what is wrong, ask, read, and investigate for yourself. Become aware of the truth.

How do you know then what the cure is if you do not know what causes your problem? It's very simple to get to the root of it by carefully paying attention to what you put in your body and on your body. Toxic elements have a cumulative effect. Every action has a reaction and many combinations. Pay attention to your actions because they will have reactions that you do not like. Do not ignore the symptoms and listen to your body and what it is telling you.

Wrong knowledge is worse than ignorance. When you are ignorant it means that you don't know any better or are unaware. Your instincts are still used to help you survive, but when you do wrong and think that the lie is the truth, you do damage. When you do damage to an innocent child or anyone else for that matter then the consequences are enormous. Become aware. Search and look for truth in everything. Nature provides answers when science fails.

Is disease a mystery?

"As a medical student, I learned about those thousand diseases humanity is suffering from. Since then, as a biochemist, I am living in silent admiration of the wonderful precision, adaptability and perfection of our body. Medicine taught me the shocking imperfection, biochemistry the wonderful perfection, and I have wondered where the contradiction lies. Anything that Nature produces seems to be perfect. Should then man be the only imperfect creature kept alive in the face of all his imperfections only by means created by his own mind?"
Dr. Albert Szent Gyorgyi, Nobel Prize winner

There are people who think that to be healthy they must be healed. Doctors, drugs, vitamins, surgery, magic chants, diets, incantations, painful postures, strenuous exercises, exotic herbs, and expensive potions have all been developed to fill this need.

It's true some of these will help. It's also true that the body knows how to heal itself. In fact except for a few genetic and developmental defects, the body knows how to take perfect care of itself. We have to give it the perfect live food first.

It is known from research that cells can be kept alive beyond life expectancy with a steady flow of nutrients and equally important, quick removal of wastes. Cells thrive when given these two conditions: **nutrients and elimination of toxins**.

Homeostasis (balance) is the ability of the body to regulate its cells together as a unit. The body knows just where it should be going and exactly how to get there.

It's incredible that everyone in the world has an internal mechanism that keeps the body's temperature at or very near 98.6 degrees. Whether you live in Siberia or Egypt, the body effortlessly makes billions of biochemical adjustments to maintain equilibrium. Through the most phenomenal of physical stresses, this internal intelligence is constantly measuring and balancing, juggling and adapting, always aiming for those common pre-set goals. Regardless of sex, race, financial status, or political or religious belief.

All who study the body closely will recognize it as living magic and that it must be given "alive" food.

We now know the body can withstand a phenomenal amount of abuse and homeostasis will maintain internal equilibrium without us even being aware of the process. If we push homeostasis to maintain order, then acute disease exists. When we develop a high fever it helps the white blood cells to be more active so they get rid of the infection. Vomiting and diarrhea can help flush out toxins. Lack of appetite allows the body to focus on cleansing and repair instead of digestion. When we are tired or fatigued, this allows the body energy to be shunted away from motion inwards to aid healing. Acute disease should quickly and decisively re-establish homeostasis.

If the body is unsuccessful in achieving its goals due to a healing capacity lower than the disease cause, then the body will slowly surrender its idealistic goals. This is the start of chronic disease.

Over the last hundred years we have developed more degenerative diseases due to environmental pollution, vaccinations, processed foods, hydrogenated oils, antibiotics, artificial hormones, preservatives and we constantly wait for future research breakthroughs to shed light on the darkness of our illnesses. In the meantime, patients are "practiced" on.

In 1914, **Henry Lindlahr** said: *"Practically all disease arising in the human organism is caused originally by the accumulation of these effete-waste and end-products of digestion and of the tissue changes."*

And famous seventeenth century English physician, **Thomas Sydenham** said: *"Disease is nothing else but an attempt on the part of the body to rid itself of morbidic matter."*

Dr. G. T. Wrench wrote in his book, *The Wheel of Health*: *"Diseases only attack those whose outer circumstances, particularly food, are faulty ... The prevention and banishment of disease are primarily matters of food. Secondarily, of suitable conditions of environment. Antiseptics, medicaments, inoculations, and extirpating operations evade the real problem. Disease is the censor pointing out the humans, animals and plants who are imperfectly nourished."*

The Father of Cellular Pathology, **Rudolph Virchow**, stated: *"If I could live my life over again, I would devote it to proving that germs seek their natural habitat - diseased tissue - rather than being the cause of diseased tissue."*

Even the master of the microbe himself, Louis Pasteur, had a major change of thought on his deathbed.

So here's your wake up call. Chronic disease is simply the inability of acute reactions to reestablish homeostasis (balance). Chronic diseases refuse to go away on their own because we don't stop putting the wrong stuff into our bodies. Your body wants to return to its normal, balanced state. If the blood is dirty and weak - a product of diet, digestion, and assimilation - these factors must be improved in order to get better health. Nobody can do that for you but you. Alive food is the best start - organic and fresh.

The word "doctor" comes from the Latin word "to teach". The doctor is supposed to *teach* you how to take care of your health, but *you* have to be responsible to do it right for yourself.

Disease is a gradual process beginning in early childhood with physical aggravation of the stomach in babies who aren't breast-fed. This later leads to decreased absorption of nutrients and increased formation of toxins that can overload the liver, gallbladder and lymphatic system. Cells need nutrients, not toxins, to run properly. So, improving health is simply a matter of improving the nutrient content of the blood while simultaneously decreasing toxins.

Proper nutrients get into the blood through proper diet, proper digestion and proper absorption. Excess toxins occur through environmental pollution, improper diet, improper digestion, improper absorption and improper elimination. When you know how to give your body what it needs then the body will heal itself and reverse even "irreversible" conditions and diseases. Think how simple it is.

Basically you need to provide the body with all the essential nutrients without aggravating the function of the digestive system. So we have to eliminate everything that hampers it, including all processed foods that aggravate the digestive organs.

We have much more energy when the body is functioning naturally without coffee, alcohol, sugar or junk food. Many people will not want to change their bad habits or accept the need for change until they experience the full brunt of major disease. The body gives us plenty of warning, but most ignore the signs. The choice is yours. A healthy body's interior is alkaline. Keep it clean. It will serve you for a long time to come.

Now you can see that removing an organ surgically will not solve your problem because you did not address its real cause. You merrily were allowing your doctor to treat the symptoms of your problem. Now you have an organ, two, three or more missing, but still don't feel good, in fact worse. Please keep in mind when you ask your doctor why you don't feel good, he will tell you that he really doesn't know what causes your problem and he will give you a drug to take so you can feel better temporarily. It might even work for a while but not for very long because your real problem was not addressed (junk food, fried food, dead cooked food and desserts, as well as stress, grief, anger, hatred, etc.). If this is making sense to you now, please reflect and let the truth in. You will be rewarded by Nature.

Many argue with the idea that we have evolved to the point that we have to eat cooked food. I beg to differ. The proof is inevitable of our health and the degenerative conditions of the last hundred years especially. Most everything we eat has been messed with against Nature's laws. Turn around and see how many people you know have cancer or other degenerative disease. Does that tell you something?

I have experienced with many people where disease is not a mystery. The problem of cancer or any other ill health vanishes when a person eats eighty percent raw fruit and vegetable diet and stops frying food and eating dairy products. What proof do we need when in Nature wild creatures have no cancer or degenerative disease as modern man does.

Even our domestic animals and household pets are suffering from degenerative diseases like modern man. They also need to eat more raw food and stay away from modern interventions, unnecessary vaccinations and processed foods like they did for millions of years.

The myth of germs and viruses

For a very long time now, germs and viruses have taken the spotlight in the fight against disease. Billions of dollars have been spent to get rid of germs, viruses and microbes before they get rid of us.

All our lives we have been lied to and taught germs are our enemy - that they're out to harm us. Some of the most clean-fanatics get sick more often than average. We have the wrong idea about germs and viruses. The truth is too simple, however, because it's human nature to suspect anything simple. We like complicated theories. We like to be smart - not intelligent. This is why we are in the soup now. We have complicated theories about human disease, and nutrition. The unique attraction humans have for germs and viruses keeps us from seeing the forest for the trees. Our life-style errors have caused us to invent the theory of germs and viruses as being the cause of disease.

Nature's first law states that all forms of life in one way or another are interdependent and in harmony and together form the "web of life." The vast majority of life forms are too small to see with the naked eye. They inhabit every space in the soil, atmosphere, water and from these forms of life higher forms evolved. Those higher forms of life depend on the lower forms completely for their everlasting existence. Upsetting this balance **just a fraction** may result in the extinction of some life forms and a drastic change in others struggling to survive. You may be wondering what part in this scheme of life do germs and viruses play? They adapt to environmental changes and always have. They have a role to play and a purpose to serve as part of Nature's master plan. The world teems with bacteria (germs) -microorganisms that form the basis for all other forms of life. Microorganisms create soil out of dead material and rock, destroy unhealthy plant and animal tissues, and actually form an essential part of the body and functions of all animals. The behavior of the different forms of bacteria normal in the body is **dependent on the environment within the body**. Plant life depends upon microbes in order to absorb the necessary nutrients from the soil. Microbes prepare the food from the soil so that the plant can use the necessary nutrient that is needed.

If you are healthy, great. If not, there are consequences. When the interior deteriorates many normal bacteria change from a benign form to a pathological one - Nature's consequence. Is this fate, misfortune, an unlucky encounter with germs of a criminal nature, or rather another step in a natural sequence of events?

What really keeps us healthy is DNA (deoxyribonucleic acid) and RNA (ribonucleic acid). Complex chemicals yet their job is simple. The code of our genetic inheritance is written in arrangement so that every cell in your body has all the DNA necessary to reproduce another you. When the cell divides, the DNA of a parent cell is divided down the middle between two (offspring) cells and each (parent) DNA always has enough information to make an exact copy of the parent DNA.

When new cells replace older cells the DNA insures that the new cells are blueprint copies of the original cell. We are finding that more and more diseases stem from inaccurately conveyed genetic information. What causes it, controls it and how?

I truly believe that it is related to the toxic environment that our body is exposed to internally by the food we ingest and externally by the pollution of the environment. The DNA does its work of passing along the genetic instructional code with the aid of RNA that controls the DNA replication. While it follows instructions, in order to construct a specialized protein that makes up each of our cells, the RNA enzymes (ribozymes) have the ability to destroy viruses and act as a therapeutic agent in controlling disease, providing that we give it proper nourishment since food is the foundation of life and life is the manifestation of food.

So is disease a mystery? How can we prevent it? The DNA and RNA must work together efficiently one hundred percent accurately if we are to be healthy. The heart of our cells, the nucleic acids RNA and DNA, along with other vital nutrients and elements, help protect and keep us healthy so that they can continue to reproduce future genetically healthy cells. As long as we allow that to happen disease will not be a mystery, but rather a lack of true information and awareness of a real cause of illness/disease. The multiplicity of today's health problems is damaged DNA and RNA cells. Processed foods and carcinogenic oils.

Who is at risk from deadly viruses like AIDS, hepatitis, herpes or others? Those who are susceptible through blood transfusions or immunizations, those whose immune systems are weakened because of lifestyle, poor nutrition, accumulation of environmental toxins and stress as previously mentioned.

When are we going to wake up? The reason modern medicine cannot cure viral diseases is that they are not caused by viruses. As **Dr. Richard Ablin** said: *"The viruses are there but they may turn out to be passengers on an already sinking ship."*

How did we ever come this far in the presence of germs and viruses without them bothering us? The problem is that today we are so run down from the way we live that our immune systems cannot handle the abuse any longer. Please read **Ross Horne's** *book* **Health and Survival in the 21st Century** *(one of the best books I have ever read).*

There is no disease in a healthy body. The cure is in the cause. The confusion medical research had in the past about viruses and their association with disease still exists today. These so-called agents of disease, like the germs of tuberculosis, cholera, and typhus, are to be found in sick, weak people, **but they are not the direct cause of the disease**. One thing they all have in common a state of diminished resistance to infection, a lowered immune system and poor vitality. How can we maintain homeostasis within the body when every function, every organ, every cell depends on correct diet and lifestyle? Disease is not caused by germs and viruses but by the wrong diet that weakens the body and the use of medical drugs that further damage an already poor immune system. Most of the germs and viruses associated with the common cold and the various strains of influenza reside harmlessly within the bodies of all people, all the time. They are a normal part of our makeup along with every other living creature. They can change form to become harmful only with the deterioration of the body that surrounds them, toxic accumulation, poor diet and the inability to absorb nutrients. The more run down the system, the more abused the system is, the more serious the infection and the naming of it. "Chronic Fatigue Syndrome" and "Acquired Immune Deficiency Syndrome" (AIDS) are popular immune-deficiency disorders today.

In reality, there is only one disease: dirty, toxic, out-of-balance, run-down interior of the body showing different signs or symptoms - a direct result of harmful eating habits, stress, overwork, lack of exercise; injurious indulgences such as drugs (prescription included) tobacco, or alcohol; or the use of antibiotics, immunizations and vaccines. Now we can begin to see how AIDS is the further, downhill, extension of Chronic Fatigue Syndrome. From start to finish, the entire show is self-generated without the assistance of germs and viruses caught from someone else. The microbes from the outside may or may not add to the problem, but they certainly aren't necessary to it.

When the system becomes over-saturated with stress, abuse, too much of the wrong foods, fatigue, the overuse of vaccines, antibiotics, artificial chemicals and other extremes of any sort, the body is no longer able to rid itself of this excessive accumulation and "dis-ease" sets in. Simple, isn't it? It may take years for symptoms to surface, but the accumulation of toxins keeps piling up until the system cannot go any longer. The straw that broke the camel's back wasn't really the last straw, was it? No, it was the heavy accumulation of straws that came before.

Our children are now paying the price for our accumulations and continue use of antibiotics and quick fixes. Today our children are being born with even more weakened constitution and poorer immune system. What can we expect for our future generations?

Take care of your body. Keep it clean inside with mucous-free natural, organic and raw food. Keep it happy, and in harmony with the wisdom of Nature. Don't believe everything you hear on television or read in the newspaper. Forgive them, for they do not know what they do. Take charge of your own life and that of your innocent children and loved ones.

Eating "alive" food makes the body heal itself

"Good dyet is a perfect way of curing, And worthy much regard and health assuring. A king that cannot rule him in his dyet, Will hardly rule his realme in peace and quiet."
Regimen Sanitis Salernitanum, 11th Century

All types of disease fall under one umbrella - chemical imbalances of the body - and all are subject to the restoration of normal health through correction of body chemistry, and proper drainage and nutrition. We have to treat the cause, not the symptoms.

Recovery is a function of the body alone, and Nature, as represented by the body, has her own ways for repairing when out of order. Our job is to assist in the removal of debris and visible handicaps to Nature's work, and to provide fresh fruits, vegetables and herbs for our bodies. Alive food has living enzymes to help the body heal itself.

Processed foods cannot heal. That is why doctors don't blame food for our ill health, or that food can heal us. They simply don't know that the food must be alive in order to heal the body. How can then a doctor teach us about our health when they don't know what causes your illness? How can they cure it then? They cannot. This is why they treat the symptoms and perform the surgeries. They want to cut out the problem (organ) but then it comes back to another organ, they cut it out again and it comes back to another and so forth. They don't want to look for the cause which by now is also due to all the damage done from surgeries. I have many innocent people who believe their doctors and have had anywhere from three to twenty surgeries without ever resolving the real cause.

When you repeat former wrong doings, wrong eating habits, it will insure a prompt return of the old problem - disease. Can it possibly get any simpler than that?

As we eat, so we are.

A History of Milk and Dairy Products

"It is good to recover from supposedly unmanageable disease, but it is better, in a far larger way, to know why one has been less than well and just how to conserve the health and vitality for the future."

Dr. W. H. Hay

(Parts of this information are taken from a Microbiotic magazine written by James Moon and John Tobe over twenty years ago.)

The use of animal's milk in the West dates back to very ancient times. It appears in both the Old and New Testaments. According to E. B. Szekely in his *Essene Gospel of John*,

"Also the milk of everything that moveth and that liveth upon the earth shall be meat for you; even as the green herb have I given unto them, so I give there milk unto you. But flesh, and the blood which quickens it, shall ye not eat." (XXII)

"Wherefore, prepare and eat all fruits of trees, and all grasses of the fields, and all milk of beasts good for eating." (XXIV)

Many statements like these appear in the Bible. However, there is no mention of animal's milk being used in feeding a human infant.

Contrary to the common belief that the use of animal's milk for the young is ancient, John H. Tobe claims cow's milk was never given to children in Biblical times. John H. Tobe asks in *Milk: Friend or Fiend*:

"How long would you assume that man has used cow's milk to feed babies? If you made the same mistake as I did, you probably believe that man has fed infants cow's milk as long as he has used milk as a food, or even since his nomadic days when he depended on his herds for what they provided. It came as a shock to me to learn that a man by the name of Underwood was the first to feed cow's milk to infants, and that was in the year 1793."

In the Western world, nomadism was mankind's basic way of life for thousands of years. The wandering lifestyle of these people resulted largely from the fact that the land was unsuitable for farming. Instead of harvesting vegetables and grains various cultures learned to milk and use the meat of a variety of animals. In order to sustain life such people had to be on the move constantly, to where feed was available for their herds. Environmental conditions are the major reasons for nomadism, and the Bible talks about the way of life that developed among such peoples. Milk was probably an important food to the nomads, **used largely in fermented form (cheese and yoghurt)**.

Contrary to the Western world, the countries of the Far East never relied on animal milk as a source of nutrition. This probably stems from the fact that Eastern cultures developed agriculture very early, and so life in these regions revolved around the growing and eating of fruits, vegetables and grains. This early development of agriculture in the East was due to the fact that the soil there was suitable for planting and rainfall was abundant.

According to the *Code of Manu*, the world's oldest human law, which was compiled several thousand years ago in India and is still the principle law of Hinduism, the use of cow's milk is prohibited, although the milk of water buffalo is used in small amounts. The Chinese and Japanese rarely used the milk of any animals. However, the use of cow's milk was introduced to Japan from China about 800 AD and continued for a short time. A governmental department of milk was even established, but the use of milk soon faded because the environment of Japan was not suited for raising cows, and because ill health developed quickly among milk users.

The use of milk products developed basically in areas of the world where agriculture was difficult. Historically, however, most of the world has depended on agriculture, even though it requires more intense labor and precision of timing. Because of agriculture, man was able to settle into communities instead of being forced to continue the nomadic way of life. This fact enabled civilization to flourish.

It is only recently in history that the use of cow's milk has become fashionable and considered almost essential to the proper growth of children, and even necessary for adults. John H. Tobe continues:

"For approximately fifty years we have been told that cow's milk is the perfect food. Now who was it that told us, or started the myth, that made us believe that milk is the perfect food? I don't know, but believe me, a myth it is. It has no basis in scientific data, fact, experience, or test. Cow's milk is not now, and never was, the perfect food for man. In fact, there is loads of evidence available to prove that it is not a good food, a healthful food, or even a suitable food for human beings.

The simple fact is that milk is big business, and as big business it is subject to the same sales pitch as any - and that is where the myth of the perfect food and 'drink one to two quarts a day' began. Please read the book by Robert Cohen *Milk - The Deadly Poison.*

American consumption of milk has indeed been very high. According to the statistics of the Department of Agriculture, the American consumption of foods per capita in 1966 was as follows:

Grains	12%	Sugar	7%
Animal	20%	Oil	3%
Milk	28%	Ice Cream	1.5%
Fruit	7%	Coffee	1.5%
Vegetable	11%	Others	1%
Potato	8%		

There was slavery in this country until a hundred years ago. When it was finally abolished, another type of slavery was introduced. The new slavery is not black but white, and now it isn't limited to the South. The slavery referred to can be found all over the country. Armed with intellect, mass media, and science, the new slavery system has brainwashed the majority of Americans, including the highly educated. The roots of this new slavery lies in the superstition that cow's milk is a necessary part of the diet - not only of infants - but of children and adults as well.

The idea that cow's milk is a necessary food for humans is a belief that makes humans dependent on cows. This view isn't new; the November 1859 issue of *Consumer Bulletin* says:

"The noted nutritionist who favored more extensive use of milk for 'super-health' expressed the view that milk was the most natural of all nutriments because it is the one thing which Nature has evolved for the sole purpose of serving as food. His idea was exceedingly appealing to some prominent dietitians and nutritionists, and to workers in agricultural colleges; many of whom were delighted to accept and spread the view that future health in American was linked to an even greater extension to the parasitism of man upon cow."

So much money was spent in advertising by the dairy industry that, according to the US Government Statistics of 1967, Americans are consuming eighty billion pounds of milk and milk products each year. This is the largest portion: twenty-eight percent of the total food consumption, and is followed by a twenty percent meat consumption. It's not surprising that these two groups of food producers spend the most money on promotion.

In order to meet the demands of such a huge consumption of milk, cows are confined, given hormones and antibiotics, and *forced* to produce milk. By the mid-eighteen hundreds the average cow yielded just under two quarts of milk per day, in 1960 over nine quarts per day. Today fifty quarts of milk per day with an average of twenty-four quarts daily. This is not only unnatural, but also unhealthy. It's not hard to understand that hormone and drug-induced milk is of questionable value. Women are routinely advised not to take drugs while nursing because they appear in their milk and are passed on to the baby. Yet they drink cow's milk while nursing their own babies.

The US Government frequently gives warnings about the dangers of milk in its publication, *Food Yearbook of Agriculture*. As early as 1959 they wrote:

"An important difference between cow's milk formulas and human's milk lies in the fact that, while the milk of a healthy mother is always fresh and free from bacteria, any artificial formula (note: cow's milk is artificial to a human body) must be heat-treated to destroy harmful organisms. Raw milk should never be given to an infant. Even pasteurization cannot be depended on to make milk

absolutely safe for young infants."

In other words, cow's milk is not only inadequate for human infants; it is also dangerous. But even so, milk consumption has increased tremendously within the last fifty years. Why?

The first reason for this increase is that cow's milk contains large amounts of protein and calcium. Because of this, many nutritionists and dietitians promote its frequent use on the old, and no longer valid, theory of high protein requirements. The second reason is that the dairy industry strongly promotes its products through television, radio and printed media. The third reason is that the daily use of cow's milk certainly does visibly develop the *physical* condition. By consuming milk regularly, a person becomes as strong, and often eventually as fat, as a cow. However, I suspect that the over-use of cow's milk adversely affects the very highly developed and more sensitive nervous system of a human being.

According to James Moon (*A Macrobiotic Explanation on Pathological Calcification* - published by GOMF, 1974) artificial vitamin D, a routine milk additive at one time, may be the most toxic chemical food additive so far encountered. He feels this artificial vitamin D, referred to as D2, causes or greatly contributes to the following diseases: arteriosclerosis, rheumatoid arthritis, peripheral vascular calcification, idiopathic hypercalcemia, coronary artery disease, cerebral sclerosis, kidney stones, urinary stones, magnesium deficiency, hypercalcemic convulsions, and etc.

Moon says (*The Macrobiotic*, No. 119, May 1977) that since the publication of his book the dairy industry has done a complete reversal on their use of D2, so that today practically all milk is fortified with natural vitamin D3. Therefore, the toxic effect of vitamin D2 may be avoided in most cases. But what of the damage done to millions already?

Cow's milk for human consumption is not advisable. Milk is highly processed, is legally allowed to contain a surprising list of chemical additives, and comes from questionably raised animals that use artificial hormones to produce more milk. It is also too high in calcium and saturated fats - which at the least predisposes one to fat and cholesterol deposits in the capillaries and on the arterial walls. Milk is a building food, and contributes a lot of excess for the body to deal with when it is not needed, as with adults.

However, I want to stress that the only milk suitable for human infants is mother's milk. The basic reasons for this are as follows:

1. Because its protein is mostly casein, cow's milk forms a large, tough curd when it is mixed with the stomach's digestive juices - which can cause serious problems. Heating it first produces curds that are somewhat smaller and softer, but still not fit for a baby's delicate digestive system. The curd of human milk, on the other hand, is soft and fine. The stomach of a breast-fed baby empties rapidly and easily.

2. The breast-fed baby normally grows stronger and better balanced than babies fed on cow's milk, even though cow's milk supplies almost four times the amount of protein found in human's milk.

According to *Nursing Your Baby* by E. Karen Pryor, "The infant uses the protein in breast milk with nearly one hundred percent efficiency. After the first few days of life, virtually all of the protein in breast milk becomes part of the baby; little or none is excreted. The baby fed on cow's milk, on the other hand, uses protein with about fifty percent efficiency, and wastes about half the protein in its diet."

She goes on to explain that this unused protein causes further trouble: "Eliminating unusable protein is largely the job of the kidneys. This may place quite a strain on a function which is as yet immature."

3. Cow's milk contains higher levels of saturated fat than human milk. This contributes to cholesterol buildup in the infant's body, with impairment of blood circulation and the related health hazards.

4. Cow's milk is pasteurized in order to deter the growth of micro-organisms. This process eliminated important lactobacillus bacteria and vitamins, which are found in unadulterated human milk.

5. Cow's milk is for calves. A baby calf weighs about 130 pounds when born. It will weigh in at about two hundred forty

pounds one month later. By this time it is already walking around. Such rapid development requires quick growth in bone structure in order to meet the requirements imposed by activity and weight. This is accomplished through the high calcium content of cow's milk - it contains three to four times the amount found in humans' milk.

On the other hand, human milk contains relatively high levels of phosphorus. This element is very important for the growth and development of brain and nerve tissue. Unlike the cow, the human baby develops its brain and nervous system first. Thus, because they have to fulfill completely different growth needs, milk for a human baby and that for a calf must naturally be different. When cow's milk is given to a human baby, physically the infant will grow very rapidly, as does the calf. However, the child's mentality will not develop at the same rate as if fed human milk.

6. The vitamin B complex, which is also important for brain function, is normally supplied to breast-fed babies. These needs are not supplied by cow's milk, especially when pasteurized.

7. Cow's milk is commonly implicated in causing allergic symptoms, due to its high protein content and indigestibility.

8. Probably one of the most important aspects of breast-feeding lies in the fact that mother's milk supplies the baby with natural immunity to what may be otherwise fatal microbes.

According to James Moon, The Macrobiotic (#119, May 1977): "During the first several weeks after birth breast milk is known as colostrum. Human colostrum contains less iron, fat, and lactose than mature milk - and more protein, vitamin A, and vitamin E, etc.

"These differences are very important in so far as the nutritional needs of infants are concerned. There is absolutely no modified milk that can simulate human colostrum. This colostrum is the primary source of antibodies available to an infant during the early postnatal period, and it has been shown that the substitution of cow's milk or modified milk during this critical period may result in absorption of allergen instead of antibody. There are additional defense mechanisms which prevent microbial invasion during this critical period, and no modified milk so far devised supports these defenses."

four pounds of dairy product per year. The amount of milk needed to manufacture the dairy product such as ice cream, cheese, butter, etc. was far greater than the USDA statistics indicated. It takes 21.2 pounds of milk to make one pound of butter.

Please read the book *Milking the Public* by Michael McMenamin and Walter McNamara. Order by telephone (312) 930-5903.

Common Misconceptions About Milk

So many studies have been done on poor animals to prove points about symptoms of diseases, allergies, side effects, etc. So many findings conflict with one another. Who did the study? And why? As the old saying goes, "He who pays the piper calls the tune." Who stands to gain from these studies? Meanwhile, innocent people are losing the war on cancer, disease, and drugs.

Let's look at a few major misconceptions. For years now we have been brainwashed into believing cow's milk is good for our bones. Truth is, milk has nothing to do with healthy bones, and everything to do with unhealthy ones. Though cattle dairy products contain a high amount of calcium, the main substance of our bones, most of that calcium never gets absorbed by our bodies because it is difficult for our systems to assimilate. The older we get, the harder it is to absorb calcium from cow's milk and milk products. People who drink cow's milk thinking they're doing their body good end up with a higher rate of bone fractures, osteoporosis, heart problems, arthritis, etc.

My mother raised nine children, nursed them all, and never drank milk. The only cheese she ate was young goat cheese, and not very often. She never had to worry about osteoporosis or calcium deficiency.

Healthy bones are built by eating fresh green leafy vegetables, herbs, and fruits. Why do you think cows, horses and other huge animals that eat green vegetation are so strong and powerful? Where do they get their huge bones and muscles? From the green plant, just like us.

Calcium in milk is lacking in other minerals. The balance and proportions have to be just right or it won't do you any good. It becomes a very complicated matter when we try to fix something without knowing the whole truth.

When you eat a whole food, the ratio of minerals and other elements is balanced naturally and is perfect so you do not need to bother with fixing things. That's Nature at work. Another example: the more milk you drink, the more you will need magnesium. The more milk you drink, the more you will crave chocolate, because cacao is high in magnesium, triggering your craving. Plus, chocolate as we know it is highly processed and contains TFAs (Trans-Fatty Acids), sugar, artificial colors and flavors. The way Nature works is so perfect! When we eat a low-calcium diet, we actually excrete less calcium from our bones while increasing our absorption of it. Just like my mother! At the age of eighty-three she did not have osteoporosis, never ever drank milk and did not take estrogen pills. Don't believe everything the doctor tells you. They don't look to the cause, they just treat the symptoms. The ads on television ruin peoples' lives.

Japanese, Indian, and African women who take in no dairy at all have stronger bones than Westerners and others on high-calcium diets.

Once the milk industry started to pasteurize milk - cook it, the natural enzymes were killed. Without enzymes milk cannot be properly digested. The pancreas has difficulty replacing these missing enzymes which causes the pancreas to be over-stressed and initiates the onset of diabetes, especially in children. Milk and milk products are also the culprits in causing heart attacks, strokes, and other problems in adults.

When the milk industry began homogenizing milk to make it taste "better", the fat in milk was spread out instead of being allowed to rise to the top. The tiny particles in homogenized milk are so small they go through the intestinal mucous and directly into the bloodstream where they become an alien substance like hydrogenated oils or margarine. The body doesn't know what to do with it so it accumulates in the arteries, joints, heart and other organs.

Worse, today they are encouraging women to drink more milk to protect their bones from calcium loss. Excess calcium is actually the real cause of osteoporosis. Milk is one reason more women are dying today of heart problems and cancer than ever before. Due to artificial hormones in milk, the cows would produce more milk and the result in women and men is breast cancer, prostate cancer and other health problems. In 1950 the average cow produced two thousand pounds of milk per year. Today top producers give fifty thousand pounds of milk. Because of the drugs, antibiotics, hormones, forced feeding and specialized breeding we also have to pay the price/consequences. Most people lacked the lactose enzyme needed to digest milk so the milk becomes toxic causing mucous, cramping, bloating and diarrhea.

Vitamin D is lost during the processing of milk and had to be added back in. Unfortunately it was discovered the vitamin D being used, D2, was a synthetic hormone and toxic to the human body. For years this information was kept hidden and innocent children were being drugged at an early age. Is it any wonder these same children today look to get high on anything and everything? The industry finally changed from D2 to D3, which is the better vitamin D the human body needs to metabolize hormones and chemicals so your bones will not be soft.

I suggest you mothers nurse your babies if at all possible, but don't ever under any circumstances give them cow's milk. And that's no bull. The XO factor (milk fat enzyme) found in homogenized milk destroys plasmalogen, which makes up nearly a third of the arterial cell membrane. Don't drink pasteurized, homogenized cow's milk. If you must have milk let it be raw goat's milk, the nearest to human chemistry.

Louis Pasteur, the inventor of pasteurization and father of the discovery of germs, admitted on his deathbed that germs are nothing. It's the environment within that is everything.

The only way to free humanity from the ravages of modern civilization is to introduce major changes in eating customs and get back to Nature. Eat living foods that have enzymes and are ready to give the body what it needs and heal what needs to be healed.

Ask yourself what might be the culprit that is causing the problem, eliminate it and you will be pleasantly rewarded. Become aware of your body so that your mind can function better and your symptoms will disappear. Milk is a major ill-health contributor and culprit to a variety of side-effects.

Most interesting is that I have not met a person that has asthma that hates cheese or dairy products. So far they all love milk, cheese, butter and ice cream. They know asthma medication may increase the risk of heart failure even the non-steroid asthma drug which were thought to be relatively benign are now recognized to have other complications such as heart failure. The beta 2 agonist are the common inhalers that most asthmatics use (Ventolin, Proventil, Albuterol and Maxair). When I insist on taking them off milk and dairy most do not want to accept that as being a major culprit of their asthma problem and most continue the use of asthma medication. But when they stop milk and milk products, their symptoms go away.

You can bring a horse to water but you can't make him drink.

If you want to know more about milk, visit the website www.notmilk.com and order Robert Cohen's book *Milk the Deadly Poison.*

Meat

At one time science supported the consumption of meat. It no longer does. The facts are so overwhelming that the eating of animal flesh is doomed as the age of enlightenment is being ushered in. One day mankind will look back in horror at the carnivorous and murderous habits of its predecessors. The eating of animals and other living creatures will seem as barbaric and disgusting to future man as the eating of human meat now seems to the average person. Animal-eating is only one step below cannibalism. Consider these facts:

In 1961, the "Journal of the American Medical Association" reported that a vegetarian diet can prevent ninety to ninety-seven percent of heart diseases.

Studies reveal fifty-nine percent less cancer among people who eat small amounts of meat, compared to average meat-eaters. (Imagine how much better those figures would be when compared to vegetarians.)

The kidneys of the meat-eater must work three times harder than the kidneys of the vegetarian.

Although meat needs to pass through the digestive tract quickly, it takes four times longer than grains or vegetables. Pasteurized milk, like meat, drains the body of alkaline and electrolyte minerals. Milk that has been cooked (pasteurized) takes more calcium to digest than it gives back! Drinking milk can actually lead to diseases like osteoporosis, hardening of the arteries, and arthritis (through the accumulation of inorganic calcium in the joints).

During World War I, Norway and Denmark could not get meat. The death rate **dropped** seventeen percent and then returned to normal levels when they returned to their meat diets.

The American National Institute of Health, in a study of fifty thousand vegetarians, found that they live longer, have far less heart disease, and a much lower cancer rate compared to meat-eaters. (Most American vegetarians were once meat-eaters and even after many years on a vegetarian diet, they still carry old dead meat or its toxins in their intestinal tracts. It takes thorough cleansing to get rid of it. Lifelong vegetarians have a tremendous advantage, even if they eat poorly, as many do. When this study was made, most of the vegetarians ate large amounts of meat substitutes, the highly processed soy products, which are also detrimental to the human body.)

In England, vegetarians pay less for life insurance.

Studies show that vegetarians are stronger, more agile, have greater endurance, and recover from fatigue faster than meat-eaters.

A Yale University study revealed that vegetarians have nearly twice the stamina of meat-eaters. (In this study, they used athletic meat-eaters, and compared them to vegetarians who did not participate in sports. Would you call that a fair study? Yet the vegetarians still won out.)

Cornell University announced in May of 1990 that "Humans are natural vegetarians." The report said: "Animal foods, in general, are not really helpful and we need to get away from eating them." "In addition to reducing the risk of heart disease, low cholesterol also protects against colon cancer, the most common life-threatening cancer among Americans."

World starvation is well connected to meat-eating habits. If Americans stopped feeding grain to cattle, the excess grain could feed five hundred million people (not to mention the land that could be used to grow food instead of being used for grazing cattle). Uncomfortable as it may be, when people see those programs or ads on TV about starving children, they should consider their own meat-based diets are a contributing factor.

When it comes to protein, people lack necessary knowledge concerning the rebuilding of the cells and tissues of the body. We have no concept of the adverse effects the digestion of concentrated proteins such as meat have on the health and longevity of the individual. The most important fact is that the human body cannot utilize a complete protein - such as the meat of animals, fish, or fowl - as an integral product, but must break it down and disintegrate it into its composition of atoms and molecules. It then recombines such atoms as necessary to build up the particular amino acids required at the moment, which may be entirely different from those in the meat we eat.

During this process of break down and disintegration, the digestive system is overworked. This generates excessive quantities of uric acid that overloads and is absorbed by the muscles where it crystallizes, forming tiny uric acid crystals in the shape of hard, sharp splinters. At this point, muscle movement causes the tiny, sharp points to pierce the nerve sheathing and the subsequent torture is labeled rheumatism, neuritis, sciatica, gout, etc.

Meat and starches are the *most weakening* of our foods. Have you noticed how we feel tired and sleepy after eating a big meal of starch and protein, followed by a sugary dessert? If they were energy-giving foods, that would not be the case.

On the other hand those who eat only raw fresh vegetables and fruits and their fresh juices get up from the table feeling energized. This is what nourishes our bodies unlike meat and starches where the food has been destroyed by cooking and merely serves as a filler (empty calories). Plus all meat is tainted by the outpouring of excessive adrenalin from the animal's adrenal gland. When we are angry or filled with fear this gland becomes more active than normal and more adrenalin flows into the blood system depending on the degree of emotion. When an animal is led to slaughter, it is filled with terror just as any human would be in its place. Its adrenal glands flood the body with so much adrenalin it becomes tainted. Then a few minutes after death occurs, every cell and tissue in the animal's body begins to disintegrate.

The custom of eating of animal flesh has been handed down to the present generation for thousands of years. I believe this practice has no foundation, reason, or excuse. Humans eventually suffer the penalty for eating meat by a weakened body and organs. This does not happen to a pure, raw-eating vegetarian. I am not asking anyone to change his or her eating habits totally. Everyone has the right to eat or live as he chooses. I am just pointing toward Nature's path. We all have to learn the hard way. You have to prove what I say to yourself and then you will know you are right and nobody will be able to pull wool over your eyes again. At least not in this subject matter! Experience is the best teacher.

The Protein Myth

Far more people are sick because of too much protein rather than not enough. Protein is in all fruits and vegetables. Though meat eaters consume more protein, they actually have more protein deficiencies than vegetarians because of dysfunctional enlarged liver and digestive activity resulting from intake of too many acid-forming foods. However if anyone wants more protein they can take variety of soaked seeds and nuts and their milk. Make sure that you pre-soak them overnight first so that the body can digest them better and assimilate them. The nuts and seeds are also acid-forming food so eat them sparingly and in the fall and winter when you need extra calories to keep you warm.

The Protein myth is myth indeed. Truly the proof is obvious. Where do you get your protein is the question everyone asks. One thing we do not need is concentrated protein from animals that puts an incredible burden on our system. More and more people have pancreatic cancer that is due to over-consumption of animal protein laden with hormones, antibiotics and pesticides. When the symptoms snowball, it is very difficult to turn things around due to the problems of multiple proportions (enlarged liver, pancreas, spleen, prostate, uterus, ovaries and other organs and glands).

Protein does not have to come from animal and it does not have to be balanced to avoid deficiencies. We are all in protein over-consumption - overload state. Osteoporosis, arterial sclerosis and kidney damage are a big problem because of protein overload. Evidence shows that certain malignancies like colon and rectal are due to excessive meat intake.

By eating whole food (raw) you get more than 1.5 ounces or .45 grams of protein a day and there is nothing wrong with that. More protein does not mean better if your body cannot utilize it and it causes burn-out of major organs. In fact less is better for a long healthy life and no degenerative diseases.

Osteoporosis

Now, let's clear up some misconceptions about osteoporosis. Osteoporosis is not a normal bone loss due to aging. It is a degenerative endocrine system disease caused by poor, de-vitalized foods that lack life force, the right combination of trace minerals, processed food that contain an overload of chemicals that alter hormonal balance.

A man in his early fifties came to see me. Before any testing I could tell he had thyroid problems. His blood test revealed a high calcium level. I recommended he get a thyroid test. He told me his doctor had done one and it came out fine. I insisted he get another one. High calcium in the blood indicates bone loss and the thyroid is the gland that signals the pituitary which in turn signals other bodily functions to release calcium from the bone.

The man's sleeping habits were unusual too. A few minutes of sleep a few times a day and no sleep at night. This went on for six months or more. An x-ray showed his bone loss was comparable to that of an eighty year-old woman. He had a huge curvature of his spine and a parathyroid tumor.

We finally got to the bottom of his problem and I'm happy to report he's fine now. His diet was drastically changed. This man ate in restaurants all his life, was a heavy meat/dairy food eater, donuts, sugar and fried foods and was never exposed to sunlight.

When compared, vegetarians have much stronger bones than meat-eaters. Phosphorus from animal protein pulls calcium from the bone. So do soft drinks that contain phosphoric acid. Too much calcium may also be related to seizures, especially if artificial sweeteners are added. Calcium makes muscles contract, while magnesium makes them relax. Magnesium is the calming, stabilizing mineral that can be decreased in availability by too much calcium. It's all connected and makes sense. Too much calcium causes PMS and mental problems in women. Too much homogenized milk is causing all sorts of problems with children, too, with their behavior, allergies, diabetes, etc.

Drinking milk, taking calcium supplements, or taking hormones will not protect you from osteoporosis. In fact, it will make things worse.

Aspirin

I'm certain you have seen aspirin advertisements on TV. Almost every person who comes to see me has been told by his or her physician to take aspirin to prevent heart attacks. We can blame this unnatural form of aspirin for many health problems we have today. Aspirin is salicylic acid found naturally in plants (willow bark). However the form used in commercial aspirin is isolated and synthesized. Look into this for yourself.

Synthesized aspirin causes ulcers due to bleeding of the intestines. It blocks production of beneficial prostaglandin (PGE1), molecules derived from fatty acid. PGE1 is found in all cell membranes. It regulates blood pressure, and controls gut mobility influencing digestion and inflammation. Aspirin also interferes with D-6-D, an enzyme that converts the Essential Fatty Acids (EFA) into PGE1. So aspirin can actually cause cerebral hemorrhage, which can lead to strokes. It causes stomach upset, vomiting, ulcers, liver damage, allergic reactions and vitamin and mineral depletion. Aspirin changes hemoglobin so it no longer carries oxygen to the brain or throughout the body. The main cause of cancer is poor oxygenation. Synthesized aspirin contains many other chemicals that are themselves carcinogenic.

Many people literally do not understand what happens whenever we do something to our bodies that is not natural. When you take something like aspirin, the ensuing chain reactions that occur within the body are devastating. The worst effect is to the lungs. Aspirin can predate emphysema and lung disease. It inhibits prostaglandin E1 necessary for the health of cilia (hair-like brushes that sweep away and clean out debris) in the lungs. Aspirin also worsens asthma. If you're diabetic, stay away from aspirin. It wrecks your over-stressed digestive system.

We create our own sickness by upsetting our body chemistry but we can also actually create health. Stop doing to the body what you did to make it sick and the body will heal itself. It is a fact that the average person who lives to be over the age of one hundred does not die of a disease. These people simply die peacefully of old age. The less medications and drugs you take the longer you will live.

Sugar - Junk Food

People don't realize sugar is as addictive as heroin or cocaine. The only difference is that sugar does not need to be injected or snorted, is readily available and is not considered a social evil. However, the addiction is just as strong. So is the damage it causes. That includes Nutra-Sweet, Equal and Spoonful, all made from aspartame.

Manufacturers are using all sorts of ploys to deceive us as to how much sugar we are taking in daily. Whenever we take sugar we change the biochemistry of our bodies and throw them out of balance (calcium increases and phosphorus decreases). That causes other mineral elements to change. Minerals work in relation to each other. When there is too much imbalance minerals can become toxic to the body. Toxic calcium can cause kidney stones, hardening of the arteries, health and immune system problems. Sugar causes a zinc deficiency and you need zinc to heal wounds. It also causes acidity in the system that makes parasites thrive. Raw food can fix all the problems, the way Nature provides.

Nancy Markle, at the World Environmental Conference on Aspartame, reported how tremendous and frightening it is as in the recent epidemic of Multiple Sclerosis and Systematic Lupus. The main reason when one of the products of aspartame (Nutra-Sweet, Equal and Spoonful) is used as a sweetener and the product temperature exceeds eighty-six degrees, aspartame breaks down into wood alcohol (methanol) that is poisonous and can cause blindness and death. It breaks down further and converts to formaldehyde. Formaldehyde is made by the oxidation of methyl alcohol. It is carcinogenic and causes irritation of the throat, respiratory, gastrointestinal tract and central nervous system. It can cause vertigo, abdominal pain, convulsions, unconsciousness and renal (kidney) damage. The methanol toxicity mimics multiple sclerosis especially diet soft drinks. Nancy Markle's report indicates that the victim does not know that aspartame is the culprit and continues its use. When you eliminate all possible causes, the cure appears. If you have any serious problem mentioned, including

Alzheimer's, Parkinson's or diabetes, keep this in mind. Aspartame is deadly for diabetics. It prevents blood sugar levels from remaining steady, causing many patients to go into a comma and die, especially if they switch from saccharine to aspartame. The products of aspartame are neuro-toxic, go past the blood brain barrier and break down the neurons in the brain. Why jeopardize your life with unnatural, processed additives? Dr. Russell Blaylock, a neurosurgeon has stated "The ingredients of aspartame stimulate the brain neurons to death causing brain damage of varying degree." Order his book **Excitotoxins: The Taste That Kills** 1-800-641-2665.

> *"Stevia - a natural plant that's sweet - was not allowed to be sold in America because it will put sugar companies out of business."*
>
> **Dr. Nancy Appleton, Ph.D.**

Today Stevia is available in the United States and is a viable alternative to sugar.

It would take hundreds of pages to cover junk food. To put it simply: everything that doesn't grow on trees or in a garden (fresh, whole, the way Nature prepared, not fried, microwaved, boiled, barbecued, or frozen) but unprocessed and untouched by the human intervention of added hormones, preservatives, pesticides, and artificial color or flavor. Think about it but don't panic. There is no shortage. There is a lot of food left.

Even mental illnesses are more prevalent today. Everyone is looking for a quick fix. It's obvious that people with a mental illness have nutrient deficiencies. Psychology was my major in college but when I realized the body and mind are interconnected - One I no longer had faith in psychology alone. I used to do decision therapy with people that worked great when the therapy was accompanied with nutrition. People with any kind of mental condition also have a nutrient deficiency (a lack of alive food-energy that is real medicine for the brain and every cell in the body). I have dear friends in California who have fostered mentally-challenged children. Their first step was to immediately remove the children from any drugs and place them on an organic raw food diet - no diary products and no sugar. You could never tell the kids ever had a problem. They all got better. In fact they returned several foster children to their parents after their mental problems disappeared. They also cured many of the foster children of epilepsy with raw food and good diets supplemented with vitamins and especially B6. The foster parents believe in Nature and natural foods. They've been in the health field all their lives. The mom won't tell anyone her age. She'll say: "I don't know how old I am, but I feel like a kid so I'll stay that way." I learned more about nutrition from these folks than from any doctor.

When we eat or drink refined sugar of any form, the effects on the pancreas are the most harmful. The pancreas injects the necessary digestive juices into the duodenum that enable us to digest several kinds of food at the same time. Sugar both overworks and disturbs the reactions of the pancreas causing it to degenerate. That does not happen with natural sugar found in fresh food.

What's so nice about fresh fruits is that when you eat them your body no longer craves candy, cakes, chocolate and other sugar-laden junk food. I did notice that people that have an alcohol problem do not like or crave fresh fruits at all. Their metabolism is so messed up that alcohol has depleted the enzymes that digest fruit so the system is no longer working properly and the body insists on acid-forming foods. Alcohol also dehydrates the body so make sure to replenish it with plenty of fluids.

Mental Health

Some of the best doctors treat mental illness with natural raw food and large doses of niacin (vitamin B3) and ascorbic acid (vitamin C) with incredible success. This combination has been used for about fifty years. Other nutrients will also similarly relieve mental illness but this kind of simple practice is no longer common today. In fact it has been completely ignored by mainstream psychiatry under the influence of incredibly powerful pharmaceutical companies. The problem? Fresh fruits and vegetables, even vitamin supplements are inexpensive. Consider the enormous cost of treating mental illness in a completely inadequate manner with horrible, expensive drugs. Add to that the high cost of doctor visits. Then factor in the suffering endured by fearful patients and their families, ghastly side effects, a shortened life span, and the failure to cure.

Let's face it, when there is a natural treatment available the psychiatric establishment will fight tooth and nail to suppress it. However you would be surprised at how many doctors, dentists, psychiatrists, and surgeons come to see me for their personal illnesses and disease. They have much to lose. But the price will have to be paid some day because we are responsible for what we do and also for what we do not do. Ultimately the law of Nature will win.

Nature is always just. This is Nature's law. We have no power to change it. This is why **Dr. Bernard Jenson** tells his students: *"I want to love you for my own good!"*

By changing the biochemistry of the body, we can change the way the brain functions too! With mental illness or any other kind of health problem, we can clearly see that we have to clean and detoxify the body as well as the mind of the accumulated debris of toxic deposits. By balancing the biochemistry of the body, the brain will reward us with good health. Simple isn't it?

Food allergies have to be removed from the daily diet. Many people with mental problems have wheat allergies and trouble with gluten, sugar, milk, additives, artificial colors, preservatives, hydrogenated oils and other things we don't even take into consideration. Parasites are a big factor too.

We must look to the cause of mental illness. Today many essential minerals and trace elements are taken out of our natural food so it will process easier or look better.

Today we do not eat food that is raw and comes directly from Nature. We spray it, cook it, artificially flavor and color it, fry it, deplete it and simply ruin it. That's why we are always hungry for more. We are eating empty calories and the toxins continue to accumulate.

There is no incentive to help us be healthy. That's why there are all the temporary quick fixes. However as you can clearly see, it is no longer working. We finally have come to the point where we have to look to the cause of all things.

Lithium is one of the vital trace elements necessary for mental health. In the past, we were able to get it in tiny amounts from real sea salt. We also did not have problems with bipolar disorder (manic-depressive) as we have today. It's so obvious that many so-called new diseases have surfaced since the alteration of our foods. Children and infants that lack the trace element lithium found in sea salt tend to be restless, sleep-disturbed, and grow into hostile adolescents and teens. Lithium deficiency is also a culprit in hyperactivity. We don't get it in our diet. Please read an excellent book by Dr. Toni Jeffreys, Ph.D. **Your Health at Risk.**

Artificial sweeteners produce neurological diseases including manic depression, panic attacks, rage and violence. Monsanto, the manufacturer of aspartame, knows how deadly it is, yet they fund the American Diabetic Association, The American Dietetic Association. Congress and the Conference of the American College of Physicians. The New York Times magazine ran an article November 15, 1996 on how the American Dietetic Association takes money from the food industry to endorse their products. Therefore, they cannot criticize any additive or tell about their link to Monsanto. Get your kids of Nutra-Sweet. "If a label says sugar-free" Nancy Markle says "don't even think about it." The brain is the major organ that controls all or functions and if it doesn't get what it needs how can we expect anything else to work well?

Antidepressant drugs like Prozac (Fluoxetine) "the anti-empathy drug" make people less interested in others. It does so much more harm than good. I have seen some who are in a rage when they take Prozac and other antidepressants. Take fresh fruits, vegetables and herbs instead. They do not have horrible side-effects. Antidepressants damage our major organs and cause other health problems. Stay away from them.

Today we have more and more people who have mental problems and depression. Our lifestyle today especially since television has a lot to contribute to it. Not only the food that we eat, chemicals that we ingest, but also the electricity that we are exposed to. We stay up late because of TV and the light bulb. We drink coffee that keeps us up even though we should be asleep. Exposure to too much artificial light messes up our melatonin hormone that can only be produced in the dark Next thing you know we are having trouble sleeping so we exhaust ourselves physically and mentally. Isn't Nature's way the best way?

Salt

Let's go back for a moment to *real* salt. Sea salt has eighty-four minerals and elements that Nature put in. During processing, all are taken out leaving only sodium chloride - table salt. Standard iodized salt is heated to above eight hundred degrees which ruins all of the natural minerals and trace elements. It's easier to handle, it doesn't clump or stick, and it markets better. You use more because you never get enough due to empty nutritional value. Chemicals are added to enhance pourability and the product is bleached for "improved" appearance. Real salt is clumpy and moist and the color of seawater. You can't pour it. So in the name of marketing strategy, we end up with a product that has no nutritional value and is harmful to our health and then wonder what went wrong with our children and adults.

We are getting sicker and have more mental health problems than ever. We are also more restless, hyper and can't find peace. We look outside for answers. Eighty-three trace elements are removed from our salt. Many like lithium are necessary for mental balance. Nutritionists and physicians tell heart patients to stay away from salt, yet every cell in our body is composed of sodium. Organic sodium is how our essential nutrients get carried into our cells. Sea vegetables (like seaweed) are a good source of all these elements. Put some real sodium in your body with sea vegetables. Fresh fruits and vegetables all have organic absorbable sodium and are the best source.

The chemical composition of the lymph system is almost the same as seawater. The physiological process by which the internal systems of the body are maintained in equilibrium is called *homeostasis* (wisdom of the body). The organism strives to constantly maintain the balance of chemistry. If there are any problems due to nutrition, pollution, oxygenation or anything in that matter, the organism will suffer and there will be all sorts of chain reactions in the body. The body becomes dis-eased - lack of ease. Symptoms then start to appear and these are what's being treated by doctors.

For more information on real sea salt, or how to obtain some, refer to the section on CONTACTS under Celtic Salt.

I'd much rather see people eat small doses of real sea salt than regular table salt that is strictly a manmade chemical. Better yet eat real sea vegetables and raw, fresh vegetables that contain organic forms of sodium.

You can imagine what a body has to go through when the chemistry is out of balance. The pituitary gland and hypothalamus cannot send the right signals to the rest of the hormone producing glands. This is why today we have a complexity of side effects that nobody but Nature can restore. Please understand this because it's very important. It is the truth. The cause of all your problems have an answer. The more complicated lives you live the more serious and complicated problems will occur. And as always one thing leads to another. Why not just realize that simple, fresh food is for your benefit and all the junk food, processed an unnatural food is a detriment.

Legal drugs

"There are no known diseases caused by deficiency of synthetic pharmaceuticals in the body, yet this is what most doctors prescribe most of the time."

Dr. Victor Penzer, MD

Modern medicine today relies on prescription drugs to treat the symptoms of perpetual wrong living. Adverse drug reactions cause hundreds of thousands deaths per year. Probably more when you consider patching up, making this the fourth leading cause of death in the US. These figures miss the possible deterioration into death of the long-term prescription drug users.

Despite the enormous cost of drugs and their side effects according to annual disease statistics, this massive expenditure has not resulted in better or improved health. The number one cause of drug addiction is not illegal drugs (street drugs) from other countries but rather legal medicine prescribed by our doctor. And what about our addiction to food additives, preservatives, sugar, coffee, tobacco, and alcohol?

Americans' health bill comes to over one trillion dollars annually. Prescription drugs account for a major portion. They are the mainstay of modern medicine, but not every doctor relies on them. Unfortunately the doctors are afraid to admit that for fear of losing their license.

A perfect example of what happens when only symptoms are considered and treated. No one wants to look for the real cause.

Some drugs may alleviate (suppress) individual symptoms, but they will not improve the health of that individual until they change their nutrition and lifestyle. And what will happen in the meantime? The famous side effects.

We know drugs are not really and truly safe or effective in the long run, but we are hooked on the idea of them. Some wonder if the FDA, AMA, and pharmaceutical companies aren't one and the same. Many think they are.

There is massive ongoing cooperation between some FDA officials and the manufacturers of prescription drugs. Think of all the drugs that have been quickly approved only to be withdrawn because of serious side effects and even death.

Doctors prescribe drugs. If one drug doesn't work they will give you another, then another, and another! And think of what happens when one doctor prescribes a drug without knowing what another has prescribed. That's when things can get deadly.

Class action suits against the makers of Ritalin, Ciba/Novartis Corporation include accusations of artificially created a new disease known as Attention Deficit Disorder (ADD) with the specific aim to increase sales of their product Ritalin. The manufacturers are accused of not advising parents of the dangers, of distributing misleading sales and promotional literature to parents and schools and violating Article X of the USPCS. "Aaron Nicodemus finds that the drug Ritalin is being dispersed like aspirin in Cape Town schools. Parents of children in the affluent suburbs of Cape Town report that their children are forced to take the drug Ritalin. Some children had been threatened with exclusion while other schools mandate the taking of Ritalin as a prerequisite for admission." Ritalin has been forced on parents, primarily single mothers. Their conclusion is that "it's easier to drug than to discipline."

Ritalin is a very powerful drug and crimes are being committed while under the influence of it, yet you will never hear about Ritalin and crime being reported. The media claims that it is a privacy issue because it concerns prescription medicine. Dr. Fred Baughman agrees that there is no such illness as ADHD and says "This is a contrived epidemic in which all five - six million children are on this drug are normal." I myself personally found that all these kids need is a natural diet of fresh fruits and vegetables, no preservatives, no additives, no fried fast foods, no artificial colors or flavors, no artificial soda pop or artificial sweeteners and no milk or milk products due to the artificial growth hormones.

Not too long ago, a thirty-five year-old woman came to see me. She was on welfare and had the opportunity to take as many drugs as she wanted without having to pay. They had her on eighteen different drugs, three times a day. She was desperate, like a zombie, but couldn't afford to see me. I saw her anyway, and told her what she should do. She told me she couldn't afford the fruits and vegetables essential for her to get better. I pointed out that the junk food she was eating - soft drinks, coffee, chips, fast foods, etc. - cost more than fresh fruits and veggies. I explained how she could plant a garden of her own in one corner of her yard. I recommended she gradually wean herself off all her prescription drugs and buy some essential support vitamin and mineral combinations until she is off everything. She complained that her prescription drugs are free and that she'd have to pay out-of-pocket for vitamin supplements. She had no clue that all the drugs she was taking were not only making her sick, they were not allowing her to think clearly! And when she told her doctor she didn't need all those drugs, he told her she did and could die if she got off them. He did not want to be responsible. Would he have been responsible if she had died from the prescription drugs? NO.

We have been dumbed-down so much we cannot tell the difference between right and wrong, the truth and a lie. That includes all aspects of our daily lives, not just modern medicine.

So many people don't realize that the combination of their prescriptions is a serious problem and more new side effects surface out of them and allergic reaction to the combination might be deadly. No one knows for sure the number of people that die from combinations of drugs directly or indirectly. Even if you don't die this time the more drugs you take the harder it is to heal the body - if in fact it's possible at all.

A thirty-two year old woman came to see me just before I left on a six-month sabbatical to finish my research on this book. It's difficult to leave so many needy people. I made an exception for this patient because I learned she was on a waiting list for a lung transplant and was scheduled for surgery soon. The woman has cystic fibrosis. She has been on antibiotics for eight years. Constantly. At the point she came to see me she was taking three different antibiotics at the same time or they wouldn't work at all. They "had" to give the drugs to her intravenously every few months in the hospital. I was amazed this woman was still alive. In fact she wouldn't be, if not for a Chinese herb doctor who was helping her on a weekly basis with different herbs and liquid nutrients to control the overgrowth of Candida, herpes and other side effects she was having from the antibiotics, aspirin and several other prescription drugs that she was on constantly. The doctors were telling her that they were ready to give up on her. They wanted to prove to her that people with cystic fibrosis die and that she needed a lung transplant. Would that really help? Then they would have put her on several extra drugs so her body wouldn't reject the lung. More pain and suffering. What kind of solution is that?

Well, it doesn't have to be that way! We needed to look into what caused that weakness in her lungs, besides heredity. The cause went back no further than to what that woman loves to eat and what she does. We immediately started to correct her typical SAD diet (Standard American Diet - high-fat, high-sodium, fast food, fried food and high-cholesterol). She was very open to my ideas and read many books recommended. It's a long haul for a person who has been on antibiotics for eight straight years. She is trying and has hopes now that she can feel better when she is free of artificial chemicals. The body always strives to heal but we have to give it the right stuff that is in harmony with our biology and chemistry.

I know there is no such thing as an incurable disease. There is however no limit to incurable patients - those who don't want to do whatever it takes to clean the body and get it back to functioning the way Nature intended. For example there are those who take advice from doctors who have no knowledge of proper, natural nutrition. Those are the ones who seek temporary fixes that only lead to deeper problems. Those are the ones who are addicted to prescription drugs and other legal substances like sugar, caffeine, fat, deep-fried foods, soda pop, ice cream, cheese, processed lunch meats, etc. They are the ones that make statistics impressive. Again it may sound to you like there's nothing left to eat, but you will see there is plenty in Nature. You don't need to give up your bad habits all at once, either. Slowly you will get to the point where you won't even crave those bad foods. I gave up bread - a task I thought impossible to do!

All medical organizations, non-profit included, have to try a little harder with their claims about incurable disease. They need to tell every member of their organization who is ill to go back to Nature and to the cause. If these organizations did that they would not exist as they do today. The medical organizations love statistics so they can put on their fliers the number of people that die from such dreadful diseases like cancer, heart attacks, cystic fibrosis, etc.

I know of a family that lost both their sons to cystic fibrosis. With no children left, their estate will probably go to a cystic fibrosis foundation to help find a cure for other unfortunate sufferers. But will a cure be found? This family did everything with their second son as with the first son they lost, down to a lung transplant. When I mentioned trying natural therapy with nutrition they said their doctor told them the condition was genetic and nutrition had nothing to do with its cause. The diet they were on would not have even helped a perfectly healthy person. The food that is the real medicine has to be a living food in order to heal any health problem.

Movie stars and wealthy people who donate millions of dollars to non-profit organizations to help save lives morally need to find out where their money is going. Just because it is tax deductible, each person is responsible to find out if so-called non-profit health organizations are telling the truth and the real cause of that so-called incurable disease. If you want to help someone, help directly with true information and knowledge and more than anything don't advertise their products that kill people. You are responsible for what you do and also for what you do not do. Good comes back to you.

I tell you this in hope that you will be more open to help a loved one in need. We really don't die, we kill ourselves with ignorance and an unnatural lifestyle. Investigate for yourself. Don't close any doors just because someone told you your "hereditary" disease is incurable. It doesn't mean you have to die. You have a choice to do what you believe is the best and most natural way. Give that body or organ in need of support, not a detriment. You will live longer and outlive that person who sought conventional medicine for help, even your doctor.

Think about this. You have nothing to lose and only health to gain. Besides how can natural raw food possibly hurt you? If you eat some poisonous plant, even then your body would just throw it out or purge it out. How often does something like that happen in comparison to allergic reactions of the prescription drugs that people take and die of daily.

We need to become more open-minded, aware, and sensible, or we <u>will</u> lose.

People can miss points that are so simple. Like what we put in our body will effect us physically, mentally and spiritually. Physically we are made of a combination of chemicals that are all in harmony with each other. Mentally we are what our thoughts are, both interrelated. One effects the other constantly, but the brain also needs nourishment in order to perform physical and mental functions correctly. Due to a lack of nourishment we become confused. The Spirit does not want to live in an unhealthy body. We need harmony.

Most importantly, I would like for you to consider something of the greatest importance. **We are living beings made of live cells that are communicating with all other live cells and their life energy depends on living food that has a life force. Simply live cells require live food to live and to reproduce healthy cells throughout the entire body that affect DNA and RNA.** How can we be born healthy or continue to live healthy and in harmony when the living communication with our cells is cut off and disrupted, unavailable due to the drug, surgery, artificial and processed food which have no vibrational energy to communicate with the whole organism. Please think about this.

Antibiotics

Candida Albicans ("monster") is a single-cell yeast bacteria that is always with us along with four hundred or more other bacteria. It is a harmless passenger throughout our lives until antibiotics came into the picture. Then it changes from a harmless yeast into a real monster - a much larger, branching fungal form (mycelia) that invades our digestive system and major organs placing the entire immune system at risk or compromise.

This is why that woman I mentioned before has cystic fibrosis. The *Candida* has taken over her body because of the overuse of antibiotics.

When unleashed by antibiotic overdose the mycelia form of *Candida* can spread to the lungs, liver, spleen, bowel, and all throughout the system. The problem is that it also produces a toxic debris when it multiplies, a toxin which has adverse effects on the immune system. It produces a substance that makes you uneasy, overanxious, and restless. **Worst of all, it can move through tissue and the lining of the gut walls, and seeps other solid elements through the system**. That causes the body to fight its own system (out of intoxication) and causes all sorts of allergies, nutritional deficiencies and sensitivities.

Candidiasis affects the whole body. Doctors don't like to hear about it because they know antibiotics cause it and those are a doctor's magic bullets of modern medicine. Quick fix that works only for a while.

If you have ever taken antibiotics you can be the victim of *Candida*. You could get tested with a technique known as ELISA. Few laboratories do this testing yet almost everyone has taken antibiotics at one time or the other. Doctors don't want to look the truth in the eyes because they would have to admit their part in the problem.

People simply cannot comprehend how dangerous antibiotics are and the damage they cause to the intestinal walls when they kill off the friendly flora. After the friendly flora is gone the intestinal walls are coated with dead mucous that provides the feeding ground for Candidiasis and other fungi, parasites and intestinal microorganisms. This is where "leaky gut" syndrome comes from, among other 20th (and 21st) Century diseases.

Now that we know antibiotics won't help you for long and that drugs are only hiding the real cause by treating the symptoms, we have no choice but to go back to Nature for answers.

Let's say that you did not take the antibiotics for that sinus infection you had. Your body would increase the fever so high that it would kill the infection and liquify it so that it would discharge the infection out of the body through your sinuses. When the body does this on its own, it knows exactly what to do. When you interfere with drugs such as antibiotics or aspirin it stops the temperature and the infection gets buried deeper into the sinus cavity where it lingers and causes damage only to return at a later date again. When that happens many times over again the damage is worse. Sooner or later it will turn into a chronic condition and degenerative illness perhaps sinus surgery.   The doctor will tell you that surgery is the only solution. Antibiotics can no longer fix the damage and it will get out of control.

The best way to fix any ill condition is to stop eating solid food for at least twenty-four to forty-eight hours (you can drink raw juice, if hungry). The body will have energy then to burn off excess debris and mucous, so the blood could flow better to the problem area where the lymph system will scoop up the debris and carry it out of the body so that normal health will quickly return. If the condition is chronic, then you may stay on this program for a longer period of time or repeat it several times until the pain, fever or discomfort goes away. It's very important not to eat anything if not hungry or when in pain. This is the safest, best and most natural way to get better and stay healthy.

Even the *New England Journal of Medicine* admits Americans utilize alternative practices more than conventional primary-care physicians. People don't have a choice in order to survive. They have to get out of orthodox medicine.

The Fallacies of Modern Medicine

Modern medicine is not working! Doctors are unhappy that people are seeking alternatives. They have their backs to the wall and know they cannot survive like this, so they fight back. Many of America's most brilliant doctors, those who disagreed with the mainstream, have been insulted, sued, persecuted, invaded KGB-style by FDA agents, and even killed. You may ask why all this for simply wanting to tell the truth and cure their patients of deadly manmade diseases? The answer is due to a lack of knowledge and greed.

Orthodox medicine and their "health care equals disease cure" mentality will not win in the end because truth always wins. John Robbins, author of **Diet for a New America** says: *"The medical establishment will get off its pedestal as soon as we get off our knees."*

Unfortunately orthodox medicine and the livelihoods of the doctors involved in it are at stake. Doctors have to start finding some new ways to make a living. The media is in unwitting cahoots with the pharmaceutical companies and the gigantic processed food industry control our daily lives. They unconsciously kill millions of people. Many more will die before the public realizes it.

With incredible media control, the doctors can fill peoples' heads with whatever they choose. The pharmaceutical companies will continue to produce vitamins they term natural, though they are really synthetic chemicals. Remember what goes around comes around. What we put out comes back to us. Ultimately each of us is responsible for the things we do as well as for the things we do not do.

Modern medicine is like bad religion. Many blindly believe and willingly die. This didn't happen overnight. Little by little people began to believe because it temporarily worked like antibiotics. Then they put too much faith in Pasteur's fallacy and the dogma of bacteriological ignorance, which he later recanted on his deathbed. *"The presence in the body of a pathogenic agent is not necessarily synonymous with infectious disease."*

As I mentioned earlier Pasteur used to believe all problems of human health were caused by one thing: an invasion from the outside. Later on he changed his mind completely. But medical doctors still don't want to accept this truth. Germs indeed seek out their natural habitat, diseased tissues, and are not the cause of disease. Dirty blood and improper elimination of debris is.

Dr. Bernard Jensen agrees, saying: "There is no disease without a cause - fertile soil."

What is the straw that broke the camel's back? When a person gets ill, it's a shock. You wonder how did this happen all of a sudden? It didn't.

Toxins are accumulative. Every day we put poisons in and on our bodies, one by one. So when a little thing happens like a cold or headache, we blame everything and make excuses why it happened. In reality the camel's back was broken by the accumulation of straws, not just the last one. In us it's the accumulation of drugs, alcohol, antibiotics, vaccinations, and invasive surgical procedures. It all loads up without us thinking about the consequences. Then along comes that straw of an additional stress to our health and WHAMMO! Some pull through and allow more toxins to accumulate. But the next time an illness happens the body's reaction might be worse and you will become more vulnerable. If it happens again and again and you keep on covering up, the outcome could be deadly.

This is why it's so hard to see a real cause. It's buried and covered up with many hidden layers of different influences of the continuation of treating symptoms.

There are many good aspects of modern medicine related to urgent care, treating accident victims and advancing new technology. However prevention and nutrition are not utilized, and thus degenerative conditions are rising at an accelerating rate and magnitude.

Knowledge is acquired by a compelling force from within, by the desire to do only good, to be able to see the truth so no one can mislead you.

Surgery

Why is so much surgery thought to be necessary? Because of the ignorance of the people, egged on by science-mad or selfish profession. It is more spectacular to operate than to teach people how to live to avoid chronic disease and operations. Medical science has not discovered yet why organs fail to function properly; and until they do scientific blundering will continue.

A young man in a hurry came to see me one day. "Like right now," he said to me on the phone. When he got to the clinic he told me no one could figure out what was wrong with him. He was determined to get to the bottom of his long-lasting suffering. When I looked into his eyes with a special Iridology camera, I noticed the bowel was very dark for someone his age. It was also ballooned and constricted in a few places. When I asked him about it he didn't want to admit any bowel problems, but the eyes don't lie. I persisted and asked him to take his shoes off so I could check the bowel reflex on the soles of his feet. With a puzzled looked on his face he asked that I not touch a certain spot on his foot. He'd had a problem for a while. He said he'd stepped on a little rock a few years ago and that the spot had felt sore ever since. Yeah, *my* foot, I thought to myself.

I pointed out the bowel reflex area and wanted to press there but he stopped me and said that was the area that gave him excruciating pain. I remarked that it was strange he was in so much pain at the location of the transverse colon reflex and advised him that could mean a problem in the bowel.

He wasn't happy with what I said and broke down. He told me the whole story about how he'd had bowel cancer. Surgeons had removed several inches and then told him he'd be fine. He was so sad and disappointed the problem was still there. I showed him how he could help himself and take matters into his own hands by changing his medication to natural food. He told me he'd had diverticulitis all his life. After listing the foods he ate, I wasn't surprised (lunch meat, cheese, milk, TV dinners, soda pop and coffee). In addition the drugs he was on weren't helping the matter one bit but instead were causing ulcers and pains in his stomach.

He was pleased with the visit and eager to do everything I recommended. A few months later he called and thanked me for everything. His only regret was that he wished he could have come to see me before having to resort to surgery.

Most people I see get better if they go back to a natural lifestyle. Sadly enough stories like that of this young man could have been prevented and his body left intact with the simple choice of living a natural lifestyle.

Perhaps people just don't realize that life is **cause and effect** and that for every action there is a reaction.

It's so much easier to prevent something from happening than to deal with surgery, chemotherapy, radiation and involvement with drugs that treat only the symptoms and cause more harm. Besides, that organ is there for a very good reason.

When you have surgery, you will never be the same again. The organ that was affected was signaling to you that you were doing something wrong. By removing or altering that organ, you will continue to do something wrong and end up with another surgery. Look at the dangerous outcome of anesthesia and removing an organ that is there for a purpose. The rest of the body will have to work harder and share the extra load. Scar tissue will block the energy from penetrating that meridian and will debilitate another organ and part of the body. Calcium that free-flows in the body will accumulate in the scar and cause a build-up of deposits. This is why I say one surgery leads to another. The worst thing of all is we are not addressing the real problem, the cause of why that organ had to be removed by having surgery, we are only creating a new problem in addition to many hidden ones.

You will live much longer if you don't have surgery, chemotherapy and radiation treatments and stay off prescription drugs. Can you believe that? But doctors scare you into surgery and drugs that treat symptoms and never tell you about changing your eating habits and diet. They truly do not believe in it. They are in cahoots with drug companies.

Here is a perfect example of what I'm talking about. My sister-in-law had six or seven miscarriages, losing every pregnancy.

No one could figure out why. She was young and seemingly healthy, so was her husband. It was a sad, sad situation. We all hoped the next time would turn out differently. It finally got to the point where she wouldn't even tell anyone she was pregnant, even her doctor. The last time it happened my brother told us her doctor recommended taking her to the hospital. She was two months pregnant but this time it was an ectopic pregnancy. The baby was stuck in the fallopian tube. If left in place the developing fetus would rupture the tube causing great pain and possible death. Her doctor performed emergency surgery and was shocked to find the real cause of her miscarriages. When she was seven, she'd had an emergency appendectomy. The sutures used caused a severe allergic reaction and over time built up scar tissue around the reproductive organs on that side of her body. Free-flowing calcium accumulated on her fresh-cut wounds and formed calcification. So when her egg traveled down the fallopian tube on that side, it could not complete the journey to the uterus resulting in miscarriage.

This sad story had a happy ending. The doctor cleaned out the scar tissue and told my sister-in-law that if it weren't for her age (late thirties at the time), she'd have no problems getting pregnant. Luckily that didn't stop her from trying. A few years later she gave birth to a perfect, healthy little boy. He is the most precious child I have ever met. I was telling him on his last birthday how anxious and excited we were when his mother was ready to bring him into this world. He was nodding his head in agreement and finally said: "Me, too, Auntie Roo." He is so beautiful and very special.

As you can see surgery can be a very dangerous business. I recommend it only as a last resort. Surgery causes more problems and more pain later on from scar tissue and often doesn't address the real cause. However surgery does work in some cases when one surgery corrects another doctors mistake or in emergency-like situations.

Always look for alternatives first and get a minimum of three opinions before deciding to have surgery. Try a natural diet for thirty days. It might fix your problem but don't go back to the old ways or it will come back.

What is health and what is not?

"There is no disease without a cause. We are what we eat, but more importantly, what we absorb."

Dr. Bernard Jensen

By now we know that health is the most important part of our daily lives. In the United States and the rest of the world disease is spreading like wild fire in a dry summer's heat. For some reason the health profession is hardly blaming antibiotics and what we eat. Instead, everyone is selling vitamins that, in fact, we cannot even absorb.

In the book ***Eating Hints For Cancer Patients*** (1994), the National Institute for Health and National Cancer Institute gave their recommendations for cancer patient's diets. Every recipe contained sugar, margarine, meat, cheese or other dairy products. Patients were told to stay away from fresh fruits and vegetables because they contain too much fiber! This type of diet could give an otherwise healthy person cancer! No wonder they haven't found a cure for the disease yet. **Or is it that the cure is in the cause.**

The evidence clearly shows we can absolutely eliminate this epidemic massacre of innocents. How can we get this message across when no one wants to hear it? If the truth were aired on television instead of drug ads touting treatments for symptoms, we would have a better chance indeed. I have written many letters to these so-called non-profit organizations telling them that there is a cure for cancer, osteoporosis, heart disease, etc. It's in the cause. I have never heard a word from them.

People ask of me "What college did you go to?" If you are not a doctor, nobody wants to talk to you; even if you are, they don't want to listen to you. I was determined to become a doctor, so I could learn what doctors know. Sadly disappointed, that was not where it's at. The law of Nature, cause and effect, not a doctorate degree. The truth I learned about true medicine was not in college but on my own will and desperation searching, reading, analyzing everything. Truth - Nature - permanent laws not germs and viruses, prescription drugs, surgery and antibiotics but a true cause.

What is going to happen to the future of humankind if we continue in this vein? What of our children, their health ruined, their brains unable to think logically and their bodies barely able to move?

Our bodies are designed to utilize only natural foods. Raw, without deadly preservatives, additives, artificial color or flavor. Toxemia has an accumulative effect and where your weaknesses are, that's where you will develop a problem. Getting drugs, metals, and inorganic salts out of the system is very difficult.

A few years ago, my son's friend was spending a night over on the weekend. For some reason, he is never hungry at our house. We offered him a fresh peach thinking surely he would like that. He said: "No, thank you. I've never had a fresh peach before. I might be allergic to it." Fifteen years old and never had a fresh peach? He told me he likes artificial peach-flavored sodas and tea drinks, but not a fresh peach.

Many kids that come to see me today really are allergic to fresh fruits and vegetables. Their bodies are depleted of digestive enzymes, so these foods are treated like invaders. They won't be able to live long and healthy lives unless those essential enzymes are reintroduced into their bodies.

Volumes have been written about nutrition, vitamins, minerals, supplements, and creative combinations of these topics that are allegedly good for certain bodily functions. What is the use of all that when we have somehow missed the fundamental boat, always concentrating on different symptoms that elude us while the evil of our health problem is the cause and the effect? The truth of anything is in the cause.

Health is something that we have to earn. Remember there is "no free lunch." Many people do not realize this until they get ill and find out how hard it is to feel good again. Especially when we look for a quick fix and it doesn't work like it used to. It causes other organs in the body to weaken from overuse, like certain antibiotics, or antacids that are no longer doing what they used to. Our bodies have gotten used to this over use, so now we need higher doses of these drugs or even have to switch to new, stronger ones, even combinations of many drugs together.

A man in his 70s came to see me who could not even climb up the few stairs to my office from the weight of all his equipment: oxygen tank, wheel chair, and a whole slew of inhalers and medicines he carried with him everywhere. He apologized for not being able to come up the stairs and told me I was his last hope.

"Please do something, anything," he said. "I am about to give up. If I could just live for a few more years to finish my work, I would be happy."

I certainly don't play God I told him, then asked why he wanted to live only a few years more. He said he was unable to cope any longer with feeling the way he did.

It would take pages to explain all he went through medically (fourteen surgeries), but he had insurance. I believe from the bottom of my heart that the health insurance industry is one of the biggest detriments to our health today. Doctors and hospitals know you are in for a parade of unnecessary procedures that can literally kill you. Many things are done without any reason. Yet they do not cover a visit to alternative therapies that could resolve the problem permanently and save lives.

I liked this man for being so honest about his feelings and sensed he would be a very good person to work with so I told him he could be playing hopscotch in no time if he did what I recommended. He would no longer need his oxygen tank, wheel chair for when he felt dizzy, or the inhalers. He was skeptical about the inhalers because he was so addicted to them. He used them all day long. The insurance covered it all. His doctor also told him he would die if he quit using them or his heart medication, laxatives, prostrate drugs, etc. I certainly did not want to take him off anything very fast, but rather very slowly. He agreed and we went to work.

Good fresh juices, lots of salads and support for the digestive system with some excellent organic tinctures. Within one week, this man was so happy he decided to try to get better without his drugs. In a three-week period he was down to one inhaler per day. He never told his doctor until it came time for a refill, then he said he'd been off all that stuff for a month - and hadn't died yet. The doctor threatened the man, and then said he could no longer see the man as a patient. And he didn't.

One of the jobs I love most is taking people off drugs and putting them on natural juices and more raw fruits and vegetables. It always works. When they don't like vegetables we juice them. Just about anyone can pinch their nose for a brief moment and drink any kind of juice whether they like it or not. I find it interesting that after a while they start to like them. When people find sense in what they need to do to get healthy, it starts to work. But many are not willing to change their addictions for any price; some even thrive on the attention they receive from doctors and nurses.

Drugs are very addictive, prescription or not - sugar, alcohol, estrogen, Prozac, inhalers and steroids. What are drugs but a chemical element that we get hooked on. And when we have them often the body becomes addicted and feels panicky without them. Try to get someone off fat or sugar and you will see. Any overuse or overdose causes all sorts of side effects, a domino effect that totally confuses the bodily functions.

Most people are involved with addictions of some sort or another. They don't even know it until they have to quit. Talk about cranky! And worse! That goes for prescription and non-prescription drugs, chocolate, sugar, peanuts, bread, etc.

During the recent war in Yugoslavia people there didn't have a regular supply of food. Inflation was rampant and you could only buy a couple of loaves of bread or a pair of socks for your monthly salary. Money was worthless. Food was rationed. Nature's law of supply and demand took effect. Coffee was scarce but if you had German marks or American dollars, you could buy it - for a very big price. Soon people were making a relative fortune buying coffee in Germany and reselling it in Yugoslavia for a much greater price.

People went crazy and blamed all their problems and bad luck on lack of coffee. Caffeine - another addiction you don't think you have until you can't get it for some reason. I was like that with bread. Vegetarians have a tendency to fill up on bread and it is one of the biggest detriments to our diet (more specifics later). It took me a long time to give up bread and wheat byproducts.

Just for fun, try to quit something you've done for a long time, even if it's something you think is good for you. Hard, isn't it?

When you train the body to do something over and over again, it just wants more. For example an alcoholic is unable to have any alcohol without triggering a craving for another drink. Nicotine is the same. Try to smoke only five cigarettes in a day if you are used to smoking a whole pack. Why not get addicted to morning hikes. rain or shine. Would you do anything not to miss them?

I'm not saying you can't overcome an addiction, but you will probably become irritable and blame your partner or family for your perceived problems. This is why eating a variety of foods is good. Stay away from the same old stuff, prescription drugs included. They're notoriously tough on your liver and kidneys. Sometimes we don't realize how many addictions we have. We basically eat the same things over and over again. That's when we get hooked. We inherited our eating habits as well as our health problems.

The more variety of fruits and vegetables we eat the better off we are. In the old days it was more difficult to get hooked on things. With four seasons you could only have strawberries in early summer. Today you can have them year round. We can eat just about anything any time of the year. However certain foods contain certain minerals, vitamins and photo-chemicals that we do not need constantly. This is why Nature provided us with variety and combinations of foods that work together well to supply the body with what it needs seasonally. The liver stores extra nutrients that we need and will use it in case of shortage or unexpected natural disaster.

In the winter we need more fatty nuts and seeds to keep us warm during the time days are shorter and nights are longer. In summer we need lighter fare when it is hot. Fruits and vegetables we digest faster and provide us with energy so we may work the longer hours that come with longer days.

This is the way Nature intended. This is Nature's law. Disease can be cured if we are willing to change the way we believe, eat, think and act because they **are** the cause of disease.

The reason we have so many problems today is because we do not listen to our bodies. We hold anger and grudges. We eat whatever we have on hand that's convenient and when the clock tells us to. Pretty soon we become addicted to the wrong foods and the wrong diet and eating at the wrong time of day. Some people eat at night too. They are lacking so many good nutrients and are depleted to the point they must continually eat more and more.

We kill weeds in our garden that have more nutritional power in them than any vegetable you can buy. Water them and eat them raw, don't spray them out of existence with toxic chemicals that later on you ingest directly or indirectly into your body.

A man came to see me one day who had just learned his wife was dying of pancreatic cancer and was terribly frightened. She was already in a coma by the time they discovered her disease. The man wanted to know not only if I could help her but if I could also help him with several problems that had begun to surface. I explained I could only suggest things he could try and that he had to help himself. He agreed and committed to do everything I suggested. Unfortunately his wife passed away the very next day at the age of just forty-two. Such a shame. Her death gave him the extra boost he needed to stay on a healthy program. He had many things to change. To my surprise he did everything we agreed on. One in a hundred. Usually people only do a partial change, then wonder why it isn't working.

We must unlearn many things taught to us by our parents, teachers and doctors. That isn't easy to do especially when we are constantly being bombarded by conflicting information from radio, television, newspapers, and magazines. Many times people come to me and ask, "If this is true, why doesn't So-and-so have cancer when he has worse habits than we do?" Sounds logical but in reality this is how it works. Besides who knows what disease So-and-so may have (and doesn't even know of) until it is too late?

Basically we all have some sort of problem, whether we know it or not. Sometimes people drop dead suddenly and we hear "there was nothing wrong with him or her." The tests just didn't show it.

Throughout history we have been inheriting strengths and weaknesses. Today we are inheriting more weaknesses because of modern civilization and medicine. There aren't many healthy people around. There are some healthier than others, perhaps, but not completely healthy. It used to be that the kids were healthy when first born but today that is not the case if the mother is not eating healthy and taking synthetic vitamins. So from a strength point of view, we are born into the world where we inherit fifty percent of the mother and fifty percent of the father for four generations back at least. Sometimes the generation skips and also you might inherit better or worse things, not just from your father and grandfather, but your great-great-great grandfather or grandmother. This is where Iridology comes in handy. Iridology is a science of the iris of the eye used as a diagnostic tool. More on that subject later.

It's very important to know where the inherited weaknesses and strengths are. With this knowledge we can help a lot more than if we don't have any other clue. The reason is that by knowing we can actually **support the body weaknesses** so that a person will not burden that particular organ even more. Powerful herbs are excellent for strengthening our body and organs.

For instance I had a lady that came to see me who had a very weak constitution. Everyone in her family on her father's side died by the time they were fifty. They all had heart problems. She told me she would die of heart trouble even though she did not have any symptoms yet. She was only forty-five. When I photographed her eyes it showed she had a bowel problem where the heart reflex was and a huge closed lesion in the heart area. I did not say anything to her other than we do have a tendency to inherit not only weaknesses, *but strengths* and that we also inherit some eating problems from our family. She agreed with me and after telling me what she ate we came to a conclusion that she would most likely die of heart problems if her eating habits didn't improve. Her family had owned a dairy farm for the last four generations. She drastically changed, now she is doing great.

Many people come with the idea that they will die of the same diseases that their parents did and they probably will if they inherit their parents diet.

Does this make sense to you? Think about it. Do you eat the same things your grandparents and parents ate? If you do, you will likely have the same problems they did.

There are many other factors involved that are a big part of this puzzle - maybe the biggest part. We are being immunized like never before. For the last seventy years we have gone so much against Nature that why be surprised at all that we are so sick. Why is this being allowed to happen? How can we be so ignorant or unaware? An imbalance in the body leads to dis-ease meaning some sort of nutrition deficiency that causes physical as well as mental disorders.

"The thoughts we think and the words we speak create our experiences."

Louise L. Hay

"There is no magic pill, only a magic process. Eating raw plant food teaches you the lessons of how to achieve extraordinary health."

David Wolfe

"Cooked food experimentation has successfully degenerated into food addiction, disease, medical science, and pharmacology. The ultimate purpose of medical science is to mend and restore mangled organs and psychological impairments, not profiteering and experimentation. In the place of medical science, raw-foodists have logic and health, the aim of which is to prevent all degeneration and to ensure a healthy, happy, long, and successful life for present and future generations. All human problems are caused by a violation of the Laws of Nature. Eating raw compels people to respect and nurture those laws."

David Wolfe

"Humanity is exhausting itself trying to fight the Laws of Nature. We are still in the Dark Ages, where every progressive idea or a great invention is for years persecuted by the corrupt few and the ignorant masses. Today it is the question of the survival or the annihilation of the human race that is placed before humanity. Hesitation is weakness. Rise up and take action. Cooked food is poison."

David Wolfe

Today people are terribly misinformed, considering the incredible amount of information at our fingertips. Despite the ways to find almost anything out, we still remain ignorant - unaware about health. We don't know how to get better. We constantly miss the point somehow. The truth is so obvious we miss it. For so many to miss it so often is tragic.

People truly do not know how good health feels - how wonderful it feels! So many people have never felt really good, so they don't know the difference between health and illness. The reason people drop dead "all of a sudden" or have only a few weeks left to live is because they can't tell the difference between feeling good and feeling bad. They've been conditioned over the years to just live mediocre lives and get by with symptom-treating drugs.

How many times have you heard of a person that you know that unexpectedly died without warning? Or a person that you know, who just found out they have a deadly incurable disease? I hear stories like this almost daily.

From the time we are born, we start off on the wrong foot. Even prior to being born. What did your mother do and eat when she was pregnant with you. Some examples are: artificial prenatal vitamins instead of a healthy, natural diet, sonograms, amniocentesis, blood tests, induced birth, and other indignities pregnant women face.

Once we are born the abuse continues. Cow's milk formulas are used instead of natural mother's milk. Vaccinations, circumcisions, processed foods, plastic diapers. Welcome to an artificial lifestyle, Little One. No wonder we grow up not knowing what good feels like.

I promised a friend of mine if he obeys Nature's laws and goes back to eating eighty-five percent raw fruits and vegetables, he will get better and feel like a kid again with incredible energy. He told me from the time he could remember he never felt like that. It started with a tonsillectomy, ear infections, appendectomy, gall bladder surgery, four bypass surgeries, back and foot surgery. After all the interventions he could not believe that he could ever feel good. But he could. He did do what I recommended and says he has never felt better. I have many people say that to me.

Please be open. You can feel better too. Just look for the real cause and stay on Nature's path. Find out for yourself. Correct your old habits, be real, not artificial in all aspects of your life and you will see the positive consequences.

Taking blood medication is not health.
Taking cholesterol-lowering medication is not health.
Taking thyroid medication is not health.
Hormone replacement therapy is not health.
Drinking coffee for energy is not health.
Drinking milk for calcium is not health.
Taking laxatives is not health.
Taking Viagra is not health.
Taking Flomax for prostate is not health.
Taking sleeping pills is not health.
Surgery is not health etc.

After an operation, you are left with two scars - one on the inside, and one outside. The one inside leads to more surgery down the road for two reasons: the real cause was not the focus of the surgery, so it will continue to haunt you; and the internal scarring causes calcium to deposit. When that happens you will have a buildup of tissue in the scarred area that will cause blockages to energy meridians. You will be unable to carry energy and nutrients to that part of the body, and other parts along that meridian line. This slowly but surely will cause incredible pain or no feeling or discomfort and degeneration within the body so the doctor will have to operate again. But this time the surgery is on another organ that has failed in its functions due to the first surgery and overburdened, and so on. This isn't health, is it?

What is health, then? Health is a state of being where you feel and look vibrant, happy, are able to think clearly and feel energetic without dependency on artificial intervention. A few of us feel that way. And you can too!

Now you are beginning to understand things better. The answers are unfolding for you and you have Nature on your side so you do not have to fear anything any longer. Not even your doctor.

I understand we all have some bad habits we can change if we want to. Remember that in Nature, **there are no rewards or punishments, only consequences**. It's up to you.

By now I'm beginning to sound like a broken record! The point I want to make is very simple: **You** are in charge of your destiny. You are responsible for the things you do and the things you do not do. What is it going to be?

When you let Nature be your guide, you can't go wrong. If you think you're healthy, just because you're alive, and regardless of all your prescription drugs, try a real life by feeling excellent. Slowly taper off your drugs and replace them with natural, organic, fresh fruits and vegetables. Watch your problems vanish, regardless of your age.

Some foods cannot be digested and absorbed because we lack the proper digestive enzymes depleted through years of bad habits. We have to start slowly, like a baby being introduced to a new food. You might have to begin with natural digestive enzymes and start with fruits which digest easier.

There are many natural therapies that will help you along Nature's path. Be in charge of your own life; learn for yourself the real truth behind good health.

Food is the foundation of life. Life is the manifestation of food.

Acid-forming Foods	Alkaline-forming Foods
Alcohol	All fresh fruits
Black pepper	All raw vegetables
Bread (Wheat)	All salad greens
Cake	All sprouts
Canned and frozen foods	Apple cider vinegar
Chocolate	Dates
Cigarettes	Dried apricots
Coffee	Dried figs
Cooked whole grains except millet	Dulse
Dairy	
(butter, cheese, ice cream, milk, etc.)	
Distilled vinegar	Fresh raw juice
Eggs	Grapefruit
Fried foods	Honey-raw
Meat/Fish/Fowl/Shellfish	Melons
Nuts and seeds (not sprouted)	Millet
Pasta	Molasses-organic, raw
Popcorn	Lima Beans
Processed cereal	Raisins
Salt	All raw or dried fruits
Glazed or sulfured fruits	(that have not been sul-
fured)	
Soda crackers	
Soft drinks	
Sugar	
Tea (except herbal and caffeine-free)	
Tofu and soy products	

Keep in mind that if you want to achieve a better state of health, eat the food that is in its original form like Nature provided, think positive thoughts, get rid of grudges, complaining, resentment, criticism and guilt, they are most damaging patterns. Substitute appreciation, fun and freedom.

Toxemia

The most common and serious form of toxemia is malnutrition (bad diet). Toxemia is due to the excess of toxic components caused by dead, cooked, and processed food. Toxemia occurs from other conditions such as stress, lack of oxygen or sunlight, infections, and ill thoughts.

Toxemia is inherited from the mother due to toxic overdoses and malnutrition when pregnant. We consider this a normal thing, a way of life. It starts with a sequence with minor infections, tonsil problems, ear infections, tooth decay, colds, flu from time to time, constipation, diarrhea, headaches etc. As we go on with our daily lives, more problems appear - high blood pressure, backaches, vision problems, etc. Then it moves deeper and deeper into arthritis, diabetes, prostatitis, heart attacks, etc. These diseases are all treated with drugs of some sort that deal with only the symptoms. Toxemia is the root of the problem, the real disease.

Where you live, your upbringing and the way your ancestors tampered with natural food while you were being raised, will determine what kind of chronic disease you could end up with. Inherited lifestyle. Many blame heredity for everything. When we inherit weaknesses we also inherit strengths that become weaker with our way of living. That will show up in new generations as inherited weakness. Toxins have accumulative effect.

Most health problems are earned and are due to improper food consumption that pollutes the body with accumulation of debris and poor evacuation of fecal matter.

Take a look on the next page, the Tree of Toxemia and find out the true cause of your dis-ease.

By changing the biochemistry of the body with raw material, we can change the sludge in the blood-body and eliminate future health problems. To do this it is very easy, you don't have to be a rocket scientist, doctor or nutritionist. You were born with natural instincts to know that what caused your problem has to be removed in order to cure it. But, you were taught to ignore your true instincts. Stop putting the junk in.

Figure 1:

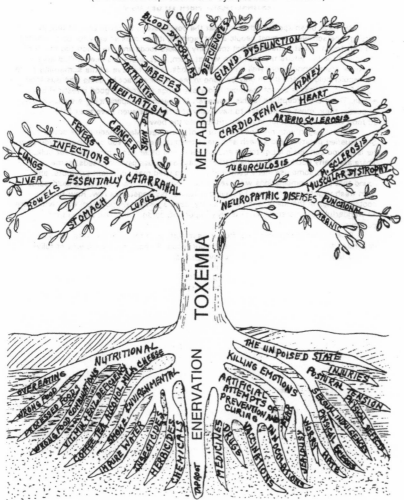

THE TREE OF TOXEMIA

(the leaves represent the symptoms of disease)

"FOR EVERY THOUSAND HACKING AT THE LEAVES OF EVIL
THERE IS ONLY ONE HACKING AT THE ROOTS."

Thoreau

by Dr. J.H. Tilden and Dr. Bernard Jensen

Immunizations

Immunizations alone have caused so much damage to our bodies and immune system that the damage may be irreversible. So on top of our natural, inherited strengths and weaknesses we have this horrible problem of immunization with which to deal. I never looked at it seriously until my son's incident and the suffering he went through. Many, many infants, children and adults die from immunization-related problems every day. Why are we so ignorant as to allow a doctor to inject a disease into a healthy baby - or adult, for that matter? Why make the body be exposed to environmental disaster when we know that we need to strengthen the immune system, not hamper it?

In the past there was a recognized link between disease and poor sanitation, poor foods, and environmental hazards, among other things. Why haven't people been informed about the modern hazards of vaccinations, or the fact that it was never a mandatory requirement for doctors to report any side-effects (including death) from their use? More than two-thirds of polio cases have been caused by the vaccine itself. German measles shots cause arthritis and encephalitis. SIDS (Sudden Infant Death Syndrome) is linked to DPT (Diphtheria/Pertussis/Tetanus) vaccine immunization, as are convulsions. Vaccines can cause a host of other future health problems as well.

The theory of immunization is based on the theory that viruses and germs cause disease. This theory has caused a great deal of confusion because it is full of inconsistencies, failing more often than when it appears to work. Too often adverse reactions occur after vaccinations. The record shows that over the years more suffering and deaths have resulted from immunization than would have occurred without it.

In the Philippines in 1918, the US Government forced over three million people to be vaccinated against smallpox. Of these, 47,369 came down with smallpox and of those, 16,477 died. In 1919, the program was doubled and over seven million vaccinated. This time 65,180 came down with the disease and 44,408 died.

The smallpox epidemic was a direct result of the vaccination program.

Read the book by **Dr. William F. Koch**, *The Survival Factor in Neoplastic and Viral Disease* (1961). **Dr. Koch** describes the disastrous increase in polio incidents in the US and Canada after the live-virus polio vaccine came into widespread use.

Dr. Robert Mendelsohn in his book, *Confession Of A Medical Heretic*, questions the safety of all immunizations, including diphtheria and whooping cough, in a chapter titled: *"If this is preventive medicine, I'll take my chance with disease."*

Richard Moskowitz, MD, says on immunizations for children: *"I have always felt that the attempt to eradicate entire microbial species from the biosphere must inevitably upset the balance of Nature in fundamental ways that we can as yet scarcely imagine. Such concerns loom even larger as new vaccines continue to be developed, seemingly for no better reason than that we have the technical capacity to make them and thereby to demonstrate our power, as a civilization, to manipulate the evolutionary process itself."*

"Purely from the viewpoint of our own species, even if we could be certain vaccines were harmless, the fact remains that they are compulsory, without any sensitive regard for basic differences in individual susceptibility, to say nothing of the wishes of parents or children themselves. 'Public good.' The issue in this case involves nothing less than the introduction of foreign proteins or even live viruses into the bloodstream of entire populations. For that reason alone, the public is surely entitled to convincing proof beyond any reasonable doubt, that artificial immunization is in fact a safe and effective procedure, and in no way injurious to health and that the threat of the corresponding natural diseases remain sufficiently clear and urgent to warrant mass inoculation of everyone, even against their will if necessary. Unfortunately, such proof has never been given . . ."

The entire concept of vaccination stems from an understandable desire to control natural processes and save lives. However the drug manufacturers are also in the business of making millions and billions of dollars without any seeming concern for a genuine human disaster. We cannot control Nature. Nature fights back. Have we really gotten a short-term gain with vaccines only to realize long-term horrible disasters and losses? Do we need to make ourselves sick or die in order to avoid "future illnesses"? Injecting a vaccine into a child is unnatural medical intervention that carries horrendous short- and long-term risks.

Parents should say NO and demand that doctors and drug companies to accept the risk rather than protecting themselves from lawsuits by asking unwary parents to sign a disclaimer like I did.

Dr. Kris Glanblomme, Editor of the *International Vaccination Newsletter*, calls for the following measures to be taken:

1) **A guarantee of freedom of choice for parents.**
2) **Improvement in the information given to parents, complete and objective.**
3) **Fair compensation in the event of vaccine damage.**
4) **An ongoing compulsory monitoring system to examine the long-term effects.**
5) **The exploration of alternatives to vaccination.**
6) **A system to deal with the secondary effects of vaccination.**

To this I add that it is our natural right not to vaccinate our children. Don't go against Nature.

Irene Allegre, Editor of the *Townsend Letter* says:

"Our species will not long survive in an increasingly hostile environment without an active immune system. Nor will we flourish as a nation producing neurologically damaged children. The proponents of vaccination consistently misrepresent the efficacy of vaccines, and the result of trials of vaccines, which show disastrous effects, especially in infants. One might wonder why there has been such a concentrated effort in the past ten years for mass inoculations of children now starting at two months of age and continuing through adolescence, when even a cursory reading of literature indicates a lack of efficiency and such serious and deadly consequences."

She goes on to say:

"Parents have been the victims of scare tactics and government bureaucrats who believe what they are told by the medical establishment."

"Active anaphylaxis is the alibi or apology of the pro-vaccination; but it does not change the fact that vaccinations are poisons even if they are 'pure,' regardless of the iterated and re-iterated process that they are innocent and harmless ... no words can describe the harm that immunizing with vaccines and serums has done and is doing except wholesale vandalism. .. The average doctor cannot think and the others do not dare to think except conventionally out loud. I do not know where to place doctors who are capable of thinking but who refuse to allow reason to guide them in their thinking in the matter of so-called immunization. Can class-consciousness or class-bigotry explain?"

J. H. Tilden, MD

Many of the children who have been vaccinated develop a variety of health problems, mental and physical, their parents never even dreamed they were linked to immunizations. We know it does. The process is not natural. Parents need to educate themselves before they vaccinate their children. I had to pay a high price for not knowing the truth about vaccines.

Call 1-800-909-SHOT(dissatisfied parent anti-vaccination http.www.909shot.com)

Whenever I see a new parent I always ask them not to vaccinate their children if they haven't already done so unless they research the subject. They become very scared because they've been told lies and that their children won't be able to go to school. Even private school!

I say so what? There are alternatives for that, too.

Growing with Home Schooling

When I was growing up we started school at the age of eight and by that time we were unfolded and at home with someone who loved us and took care of us dearly. Maybe we didn't learn how to read at the age of three but we learned a lot about life's routines.

Inventor Thomas Edison was told he wasn't fit for school. Genius Albert Einstein was a so-so student. Kids would be better off home-schooled or tutored by someone that genuinely loves kids without being brainwashed and lied to by some teachers or exposed to school cafeteria foods, soda pop, candy bars, homogenized artificially-flavored chocolate milk, and other horrible things. Who can forget the flap caused a few years ago when one school district wanted to designate catsup a vegetable?

When my youngest son was in third grade the teacher asked the class to read a book of fiction, and then write a report. I called the teacher and asked him if my son could do a report on a non-fiction book about Nature or reality. The teacher said absolutely not. He'd been teaching third-grade for fifteen years and I was the only parent who ever "complained". I then called the school principal and spoke with him about how I felt about Nature and reality and how that should be in everyone's interest. The principal too, disagreed because he didn't want to change curriculum. I told him if that was all the better he could do, I'd be happy to take my son out and place him back in the private school he'd just come from the previous year. The principal realized I was adamant about what books my son should be allowed to read, and finally gave in.

I knew my son would pay a high price for going against the system but we went ahead because the school year only had a few months left to go.

The teacher sent home a flyer outlining what was expected in the book report. My son did a report in complete accordance with the flyer. It took him many, many hours, and at the end of the report he drew a beautiful picture. The drawing also took many hours, but it was required by the teacher. I was impressed with my son's effort and gave him an A+. I also told him not to expect that high a grade from the teacher.

A few days went by and then my son came home in tears, went to his room and said he would never go to school again. He told me of thirty kids in the class, he'd received the absolute worst grade on his book report. He begged me to call the teacher immediately. He was devastated!

I called and asked the teacher what was going on. He wanted to meet with me the next week to discuss the matter. I said it was much too important to wait because my son refused to leave his room or to ever go to school again. This was serious. I asked what my son had done to deserve the lowest grade in the class. The teacher told me my son had done a full book report when all he'd been asked for was a partial. He told me that because my son didn't listen to his instructions, he was penalized. Never mind the fact that this teacher had sent home written instructions I double-checked myself to make sure my son had followed them to the letter.

I was shocked. What kind of lesson was this? When you do more and better you are punished. No wonder children grow up so confused. I realized then further argument would be useless. The system - and this teacher's mind - was set in stone. Needless to say, we made the decision right for us, and my son never set foot in public school again.

A love for learning never asks what grade you are in. Kids are born with a burning desire to seek knowledge but school is not a place for learning. School has become a place for baby-sitting and brainwashing our children. The education system starts kids early filling their innocent heads with half-truths based on hidden agendas that take a lifetime to unlearn.

Schools are too stressful today even dangerous at times. I suggest if you have children or want to have them, you'd best take matters into your own hands or you might be unpleasantly surprised. For the sake of our kids' future health and sanity rely on your natural parental instincts. Schools are not what they used to be. They separate all ages into same age groups yet they don't communicate enough. The peer pressure is enormous.

There are still many teachers who are excellent and love what they do. You will always remember those as your mentors.

They themselves are unhappy with curriculum that is forced upon them. Many teachers feel bad for the kids.

I have heard many excuses why parents send their children to school but not one makes sense in the larger scheme of life. The need for a child to socialize is the biggest excuse, despite the fact children are severely limited as to the time actually spent socializing while attending school. Think about how unnatural it is to send a toddler to daycare with some stranger. There are times when a parent, especially a single parent, must rely on daycare in order to put food on the family table. How sad to think situations like this rarely happened in the past, when several generations of a family lived together. Our society has gone against Nature and become fractured to the detriment of our future - our children.

Why does the government legislate the installation and wearing of seat belts for passenger vehicles, then allow our children to be transported to and from school in buses without seat belts? They ruin our children's immune systems with mandatory vaccinations for school and universities, then punish the child by keeping them out of school if the parent chooses not to allow the vaccines. What ever became of parental rights? Demand them back. You have a choice. Sign a waiver. Stand up for what's right. Stand up for Nature.

Children don't need to be in a learning environment where they are bossed around all day, where they learn to compete instead of get along, where being better is more important than being yourself. A place where intolerance for difference is fostered and where you are lied to, usually by omission. Where the wrong kinds of knowledge are emphasized over the common sense required to make it through life on your own. There are always exceptions, but too few and far between.

Read the book *All I Ever Needed To Know I Learned In Kindergarten,* by Robert Fulgrum. Or the one by James W. Loewen, *Lies My Teacher Told Me.* These and other books are in the Suggested Reading at the end of this book.

When I was growing up, my dream was to learn how to read so I could teach myself what I wanted to know without having the knowledge being filtered through someone else's interpretation.

It wasn't until I got out of college though that my true learning began. Until then it was theory after theory, statistic after statistic, and the memorization of useless nonsense I promised myself to forget after final exams. I can honestly say that we learn only what we are interested in and all that other stuff is a chore that takes years off your life. We teach ourselves. The teacher will appear when the student is ready, not when someone else thinks you should be.

Most teachers do the absolute best they can, the best they know how to do. Unfortunately they often don't know what is best for our children and their future.

We are all individuals; we do our own things when we are ready - physically, mentally, spiritually and emotionally. That's healthy!

One of the biggest reasons why I'm writing this book is to help our children, schools and colleges to teach children about Nature and true nutrition. Every chance I have, I go to different cities and talk to principals and teachers about our future generation. When I hear all the problems that are going on in schools it's easy for me to see that they always revert to the cause, but they don't see it somehow. How they feed our kids literally with food and thoughts is the key. I'm making some progress and will not stop. The road is rough but it is the future of our new generations and our responsibility.

We need more volunteers. Many teachers have been helping tremendously even though their hands are sometimes tied. Only with persistence and true knowledge can we bring the awareness into our schools.

What is the Point?

There comes a time when you wonder what is the point in all the mysteries of health and illness. What is good for this problem or that problem? Quick fixes do not work. You no longer know who to listen to or whom to believe. Everyone is pushing their "cure." New discoveries surface for every imaginable problem yet the suffering we are facing today is worsening.

The fact is that in order to get rid of any so-called disease we have to get rid of toxemia (sludge, dirty, sticky blood, debris and bad thoughts) because it is this state of blood, bad thoughts, etc. that makes disease possible. Infections, drugs and food poisoning may kill us, but if they do not, they will be short-lived in the subject free from enervation and toxemia. In fact, the poisoning will continue and linger in the system until toxemia is overcome so the elimination channels can remove all the traces of the infection and debris.

I'm at the point right now, totally saddened, wondering whether we are ever going to wake up to the simple truth-fact that the cure is in the cause. Nothing else matters or will ever change until we understand that simple truth.

So the point is how long are we going to continue to hide the truth (cause and effect) and continue to suffer and die? Yet it would be so simple to embrace the truth and bring the awareness into every being so that our future could change forever, finally freeing all humanity of dogma, disease and quick fixes. How can we do it? How can we get this point across?

We need volunteers. We are trying to help with free seminars on cooking/uncooking classes, talks on the radio and television as well as schools. Any ideas are welcome. Please stay in touch and keep checking our website. Together we can succeed and help save the innocent ones. My point is not to force anyone to change, but rather to make true knowledge available to all that want it, so they can decide for themselves what is best. Please let us know if your organization would be interested in a lecture or seminar.

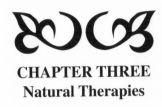

CHAPTER THREE
Natural Therapies

"First, do no harm."
Hippocratic Oath

The validity of any healing treatment can only be judged by the individual complete return to well being. The individual is the key, because each and every one of us has certain inherited weaknesses that have to be addressed and strengthened in the safest, most complete way possible without deteriorating the condition further. We are not a statistic.

Many people today are questioning conventional medical wisdom and realizing it is not always the right thing to do. It does not address the *real* problem. The situation of a patient usually worsens or produces more symptoms due to the fact that the real cause of the problem isn't being addressed. If you've read the previous chapters of this book, by now you know how to look for the real cause and restore health to harmony and balance.

There are many natural therapies available to make a patient feel better with the least harm done to the individual. Disease is the outward manifestation of inner disharmony. Symptoms are signs of deeper imbalance. It is very important to relieve the symptom and reach the root of the problem or cause. The key is to explore and consider the deeper hidden problems.

In any natural therapy, nutrition is key. Proper nutrition will help bring a problem to an end faster than any therapy alone or combined. Raw food and juicing are the keys.

Fasting is sometimes the best way to heal the body that has been overburdened by too much toxic waste and the wrong kinds of foods. Stopping the intake of any food shows positive results so that the blood can circulate quicker and better to the area of need. See books on fasting listed in the SUGGESTED READING.

There are three main points to consider with natural therapies:

1) Look for the main problem of the individual, whether physical, emotional or mental.
2) Look at the person as a whole. We cannot divide the person into parts to be treated separately. Consider every complaint.
3) Select the best treatment available for the individual, not just for the complaint. And always pay attention to food first.

Stress plays a major role in disease and can be analyzed from different directions. Many therapies combined can help alleviate stress. Stress has many different manifestations: physical, emotional, and mental. It can even be all three together. Though stress plays a negative role in our lives, we need to recognize it, learn how to cope with it, reduce it and simply relax. So many different therapies can be utilized to help a person get better.

Many therapies are included in the following pages.

Following is a list of the some of the most widely used natural therapies:

• Alternative Medicine • Aroma Therapy • Naturopathy •
• Chinese Medicine • Nutritional Therapy • Iridology •
• Acupuncture • Reflexology • Acupressure • Kinesiology •
• Herbology and Herbal Medicine • Flower Therapy and Remedies•
• Homeopathy • Chiropractic • Osteopathy • Hypnotherapy •
• Psychotherapy • Focusing • Massage • Body Work •
• Hands-on Healing • Qi Gong • Shiatsu • Hydrotherapy •

There are many more. All of these therapies can do wonders for people with various conditions, however Naturopathy and nutrition need to be included in any therapeutic programs to assure better health and faster recovery. The easiest way to get to the point and the heart of the problem is by eliminating all possible causes one at a time.

Naturopathy

"Let food be your medicine and let medicine be your food. Only nature heals, provided it is given the opportunity."
Hippocrates, 500 BC

Natural medicine, or natural hygiene, is a term covering that self-healing mechanism of the body which is automatically in harmony with Nature. For eons, man has used nature to heal himself, more often by accident than by design. Naturopathy means the healing qualities of Nature as used in the past. Fasting was often used to give the body a chance to rest and throw off or burn up toxic wastes and mucous. Different plants, herbs and foods were known to revitalize and strengthen various organs and systems of the body, as seawater, hot springs, mud baths, and rivers have long been used to relieve aches and pains, and help restore vitality and vigor. The peace and calm that comes from relaxation and meditation have been known and practiced by many ancient cultures. A movement is in force today returning us to these simple truths of Nature.

In the past man's health depended on being in harmony with Nature and the Universe through the use of natural elements such as air, sunlight, water, food, herbs, movement and rest to regain health.

Over the last two centuries, many lost touch with these simple ideals. We have become a more industrialized, modernized, and suburbanized society with a food and water supply increasingly poisoned and polluted. Our diet is far removed from the fresh, natural raw vegetables, fruits, nuts, seeds of our ancestors. Many people eat meat two or three times a day. Today it is over-refined and chemically tampered with, we eat too much of it and we don't earn our food through hard labor like we used to. In fact ninety-five percent of people eat mainly cooked food that has no life force left in it. How can people expect to be vibrant and energetic on a diet such as this?

There are positive sign however that people are growing more aware of the negative effects of such a lifestyle and are looking for alternate methods of combating these problems via an increasing demand for organic whole foods and the support for the ecological movement.

Naturopathy is founded in the importance of the body's natural vitality that leads it toward self-cleansing, self-repairing and self-healing. This built-in mechanism works on its own if nothing is impeding the process.

The body is well equipped by Nature to withstand various internal changes, such as hormonal regulation during the menstrual cycle, and external ones like the changing seasons. We have an excellent defense system that has evolved over the centuries, but we expose ourselves to all kinds of abuses: poor posture and muscle tone from sitting for long periods of time or from lack of exercise leading to poor circulation and the accumulation of wastes; use of drugs that mask symptoms and lead to unwanted side-effects; the excessive use of stimulants; occupational or environmental hazards such as asbestos, lead, formaldehyde, or plastics in our homes, carbon dioxide in our air, or chloride, fluoride, phosphorous and detergents in our water. All these factors and more break down our defenses and lead to disease. In addition, eating lifeless food cannot heal a living body.

The body has ways to free itself of disease the result of which ultimately strengthens the body. Although these can be unpleasant, they are the body's way of reestablishing health and are to be **encouraged** rather than suppressed. Let the catarrh/debris/ toxins out at any price. Never take drugs to suppress it.

First the body develops a fever that increases the metabolic rate and circulation of blood and lymph thus speeding the removal of toxins. A raised temperature also creates a less-favorable environment for bacteria. Therefore in naturopathic treatment it is important to let the fever run its course. The acute discomfort experienced with a cold is necessary to remove toxins from the body. As irritants, bacteria and viruses stimulate the production of secretions toward the nearest exit. Toxins turn into liquid forms (discharge) so they can be easily expelled.

If we do not allow this acute condition to proceed, then waste accumulates within the body and becomes toxic, eventually destroying tissues and organs, driving the toxic material deeper and making it much more difficult to expel. This leads to a chronic condition much harder to treat.

The second principle of Naturopathy concerns the nature of disease, the manifestation of the vital force trying to rid the body of any obstruction to proper function. The Naturopath tries to discover whether the cause is chemical, mechanical, or psychological in so far as we can separate these factors that influence one another.

A chemical cause of disease would mean an excess of waste products due to poor kidney, lung or bowel function, or poor circulation of bodily fluids such as lymphatic due to dietary deficiency or dietary excess.

A mechanical imbalance can be due to poor posture caused by a sedentary lifestyle. This can lead to spinal tension, the malfunctioning of the entire area around the vertebrae so the nerves, blood supply and lymphatic circulation are affected.

A psychological cause refers to the particular characteristics of the individual and how he or she is affected by stress situations in any and all parts of life.

The Naturopath again is concerned with the whole body in its environmental context. The unique response of each individual to that environment is fundamental to the way a Naturopath treats a patient. So the Naturopath takes into account the entire person, trying to find the cause of an illness as opposed to simply dealing with symptoms. The **Cure** lies in the **Cause**. We must remove any possible cause.

Naturopathy treats the person as a whole. There are few conditions that cannot be treated by Naturopathy given a commitment to health on the part of the individual. As a general rule you can consult a Naturopath about the same complaints you'd take to your General Practitioner. The Naturopathic Doctor (ND) would send you for further tests if he or she suspects a pathology or fracture.

Naturopathy compliments many other alternative therapies and provides an excellent foundation for good health. It gives the individual back the responsibility for his or her own treatment and by using other therapies like herbal therapy, reflexology, psychotherapy, acupuncture, homeopathy, osteopathy, or massage.

A person can make changes in his/her life in the areas of rest, exercise, diet, fasting, hydrotherapy, relaxation, and common sense natural treatments. Naturopathy incorporates a good balance of air, sunlight, movement and water with nutrition.

The Naturopath will be interested in your family history of disease so he/she would be able to strengthen the weaknesses. If such a history exists, this will increase your ability to overcome a particular complaint. Your body type will guide the ND to the kind of diet that will suit you. No drugs, just supporting the entire body. With natural food the body will heal even the "incurable".

This is why I chose Naturopathy. It made so much more sense to look at the whole person, always concerned with the cause of the problem not just the symptom.

When you explain this to an ill person, it makes sense and it's easy to get them to see all the steps of their problem unfold. When they begin to feel better, they get more encouraged to take care of themselves and be in charge of their own health. The choice is theirs.

Eating of natural food in their original raw form has been taking place since the beginning of time. This is not new dogma. Only since the rediscovery of fire did humans start to cook and process their food. *"If you look at the clock and compare it to how long humans have been eating cooked food since the beginning of time, it would come out to about five seconds."*

Look how much damage it has done to us especially the last sixty years. Why do you think we have all the modern man diseases - cancer, arthritis, heart disease, etc. When you incorporate all the other damage we have been doing to our food (genetic engineering, pesticides, environmental toxicity to our body and the planet, vaccines, flu shots, surgery, radiation, chemotherapy, etc.) you can see how we have to go back to Nature. We have strayed away and we are paying for it.

Nutrition Therapy

"You cannot prevent birds of sorrow from flying over your head, but you can prevent them from building nests in your hair."
Chinese proverb

We Are What We Eat

Nutrition therapy is as old as medicine itself. Right up to modern times doctors have always told their patients what and what not to eat. Only since the advent of "wonder drugs" has nutrition become no longer fashionable as a form of treatment, except under rare circumstances. Nutrition therapy, as it's practiced today began in the early days of Naturopathy during the late nineteenth and early twentieth centuries. J. H. Kellogg, Vincent Priessnitz, and Sebastian Kneipp were some of its early pioneers. The movement used nutrition and fasting together with other therapies to cleanse the body and build up its self-healing ability.

We've learned a lot since those days of how the body works: hormones, enzymes, blood and cells themselves. We have learned more about the composition of food, vitamins, and essential fatty acids. We know more how they are broken down or metabolized, how they combine and interact with other nutrients to nourish specific bodily functions. We know more about amino acids, the building blocks of protein, how they knit together in enormously complex patterns with other nutrients to produce everything our body is made of.

Specialist practitioners of nutrition therapy, at first only doctors, began to emerge in the 1950's, using this new knowledge to devise diets and regimens of vitamins and minerals specially targeted at specific symptoms and various illnesses. Nutrition therapy thus became a much sharper tool with a scientific basis. This therapy has been developed and fine-tuned over the years and is now a highly-sophisticated health care system which uses knowledge of physiology and body chemistry to explore all ways of manipulating a patient's nutrition to achieve a desired therapeutic effect. Some Naturopaths incorporate advanced nutrition therapy into their treatments but this depends very much on the individual practitioner and circumstances.

Therapy depends on the broad diagnosis of an individual:

1)   An allergy or sensitivity to a food or to something in the air or environment.

2)   Toxic overload due to heavy metals or chemicals in the environment. Lack of efficiency in eliminating waste products from the body or poor liver action.

3)   Nutrition deficiencies due to poor diet, special needs or poor absorption.

One thing modern nutrition missed is the fact that the body will not be able to totally heal itself if it is not given alive food that carries live enzymes and life energy. Raw organic food is real medicine without side effects (**Cure**). Doctors today do not believe in food having anything to do with our diseases or curing anything because processed/cooked food does not get people well. Only raw food can be healing to a toxic ill person and restore the body to health.

Many problems affecting the skin, moods, sinuses, and digestive system, among others, are caused by eating something that "disagrees" with you. This includes common foods such as coffee, bread or sugar. Sometimes symptoms may not surface immediately after eating but can be delayed or appear only occasionally, usually when under stress.

Toxic overload, particularly as age advances causes problems due to internal pollution or lack of efficiency in eliminating waste products from the body properly and not often enough. These waste products can cause fatigue, fluid retention, arthritis, skin problems, re-absorption of toxins, and other symptoms as they block and poison the body's processes.

Nutritional deficiencies are common if your eating habits are not what they should be or if you are not assimilating/absorbing all the nutrients from your food. You may have slight deficiencies that could affect your skin, nerves and hormones in particular. Due to poor absorption it is possible to have symptoms of nutritional deficiency even if you eat a healthy balanced diet. This is why a nutritional therapist often makes use of dietary supplements. The problem is that supplements can be made of cheap synthetic chemicals that are poorly absorbed and are ill designed to correct deficiency symptoms. Some multivitamin and mineral products may lack a number of nutrients and even make the body worse by leaching out essential nutrients and elements. Proper nutrition and absorption is the key. Eat lots of organically grown fresh fruits and vegetables to keep the body free of mucus and blockages.

Nutrition therapy is all about exploring how an individual's health has gone wrong and helping that person understand how to put it right by using nutrition and a better knowledge of the body to make certain it does not happen again. Nutrition is the most essential of all therapies. If your nutrition is not right it is likely other treatments will fail. Every part of your body is made from what you once ate. Food is the foundation of life and life is the manifestation of food.

Every patient comes to nutrition therapy after years on homeopathy, acupuncture or any other therapy complaining that these treatments only seem to work for a limited period. Once a treatment ceased, the problem returned. These patients have nutritional imbalances that other therapies helped alleviate to a point but could not cure.

Remember, we are what we eat and what we can absorb.

In order to understand nutrition we have to know the processes the foods we eat must go through to be digested and become nourishment for the cells and tissue in our body as well as poisons that we must eliminate or fight off.

If we taught the study of human anatomy in elementary school children would learn the importance of their body and that when properly nourished as Nature intended it to be, they would develop into much more intelligent beings because their faculties would be more alert and clear. They would discover there is nothing mysterious in the cause of sickness and disease, and that Nature has furnished us with all the means to prevent illness throughout our life. The children would learn to grow with an appreciation of all life and grow to love and respect, not injure, animals or other human beings. Instead children are taught in school how to be "smart." Smart for what? Memorizing dates, the current take on history and phony-baloney knowledge or theories that make no sense whatsoever?

If we were trained from childhood to understand the functions of our body, we would know that our body is composed of millions of microscopic cells. They compose all the tissues, the liquids, and the bones in our system. Microscopic as they are, they are nevertheless endowed with life and intelligence. They respond to the stimulus of the mind, whether we are conscious of this or not. They are our *servants* in every conceivable respect. They must have nourishment in order to carry on their work. We must give it living foodstuff - living vibrant energy. No one can work and live if they are starving. Most importantly, the quality of their work is directly related to the quality and quantity of the food they are allowed to have. More doesn't mean better, even if it's the best stuff. In fact less is more.

Nature has endowed our bodies with tolerance in regard to the care that we give to our cells. When the limit of such tolerance has been reached we are warned in an indirect manner through tiredness, fatigue, headaches, pains and aches. If we ignore these warnings, Nature stops us with sickness or disease. Consequences. This happens because of the environment of the cells and their nourishment or if we failed to cleanse the body of accumulated waste (poisons the cells absorbed from accumulated debris in the system). So the nourishment for the little cells must be vital and alive and it must be of such a nature that the digestive processes can separate and segregate the atoms and molecules composing it so that the blood stream and the lymph can carry them to their cells and out.

It is our duty to understand this principle of cell nourishment and teach our children from the beginning the truth about live food (as opposed to dead, processed and cooked food) for the care of the cells and tissues in our body system. The vegetables and their juices are the builders of the body and fruits and their juices are the cleansers of our cells in the body. They also must be raw in order to be vital and of constructive value. When they are processed, preserved or pasteurized, their life principle has been destroyed. Is this taught in medical schools and nutrition classes?

Atoms and molecules are some of the smallest particles into which matter can be broken down. So vegetables and fruits are composed of atoms and molecules. When two or more atoms are joined together they become a molecule. The chemical formula of water is H2O, meaning that the smallest particle of water is composed of two atoms of hydrogen and one atom of oxygen. Raw fruits and vegetables are loaded with water and oxygen.

The formula of the starch molecule is C6H10O6, meaning it's composed of six atoms of carbon, ten atoms of hydrogen, and six atoms of oxygen. Interestingly enough the starch molecule is not soluble in water, alcohol, or ether. This is why grains and starchy foods eaten in large quantities cause impaction in the liver, stones to form in the gallbladder and kidney, why the blood coagulates in the blood vessels and capillaries, and forms all sorts of trouble: tumors, cancer, hemorrhoids, and many other disturbances throughout the system.

Because the starch molecule is not soluble in water it travels throughout the blood and lymph systems as a solid molecule that cells, tissues and glands of the body cannot utilize, so the body tries to expel it. When the elimination organs become afflicted with all the accumulation of these molecules as a lining of their walls (like plaster on the walls of a room) they cannot be expelled through these channels. They look for other exits in the form of allergies, high blood pressure, cancer, etc. No system of healing can be permanently effective until the eliminative organs have been thoroughly cleansed of accumulated waste matter, and simultaneously all grains and starchy foods expunged from the diet. Raw food is mucous free.

When we eat sugar in any non-natural form it ferments in the system causing the formation of acetic acid, carbonic acid, and alcohol.

Acetic acid is a powerful destructive acid as witnessed by its use to burn warts off the skin. You can imagine what it does to the delicate membranes in the intestinal tract. It rapidly penetrates the system and because of its affinity for the fats in the nerve texture it reacts on the nerves with paralyzing consequences.

Alcohol is worse. It acts as a solvent for vital elements in the brain, kidneys, liver and nerves. Elements in the body that are only soluble in alcohol are very difficult to rebuild.

However when we eat or drink refined sugar of any form the effects on the pancreas are the most harmful. The pancreas injects the necessary digestive juices into the duodenum that enable us to digest several kinds of food at the same time. Sugar both overworks and disturbs the reactions of the pancreas causing it to degenerate. That does not happen with natural sugar found in fresh food.

When it comes to protein, people lack necessary knowledge concerning the rebuilding of the cells and tissues of the body. We have no concept of the adverse effects the digestion of concentrated proteins such as meat has on the health and longevity of the individual. The most important fact is that the human body cannot utilize a complete protein - such as the meat of animals, fish, or fowl - as an integral product, but must break it down and disintegrate it into its composition of atoms and molecules. It then recombines such atoms as necessary to build up the particular amino acids required at the moment, which may be entirely different from those in the meat we eat.

During this process of breaking down and disintegration, the digestive system is overworked. This generates excessive quantities of uric acid that overloads the system and is absorbed by the muscles where it crystallizes, forming tiny uric acid crystals in the shape of hard, sharp splinters. At this point, muscle movement causes the tiny, sharp points to pierce the nerve sheathing, and the subsequent torture is labeled rheumatism, neuritis, sciatica, gout, etc. Taking drugs for this problem does not work. You must remove the cause.

Meat and starches are the *most weakening* of our foods. Have you noticed how we feel tired and sleepy after eating a big meal of starch and protein, followed by a sugary desert? If they were energy-giving foods, that would not be the case.

Germs and bacteria were created by Nature to break down and disintegrate waste matter. They are not in the least bit harmful in and of themselves. It is their by-products, the sewage of their colonization in the presence of excessive putrefaction that causes the trouble.

In the preparation of our meals, every food present represents a chemical combination of elements, atoms, and molecules, according to a plan of Nature. When the foods are composed of raw vegetables and fruits, the elements composing them are vital, organic, live elements and can be combined in any desired mix. Any such mixture is advantageous. The elements combine in a natural manner making the result beneficial.

However when foods are processed or cooked, the elements composing them have become de-vitalized and their original chemical composition changed. This applies to all foods.

Starches, grains, and sugars create an acid reaction in the body when eaten. In the process of digestion they require the action of the alkaline digestive juices.

Concentrated proteins such as meats, fish, fowl, eggs, and dairy products; belong to the acid category and require the acid digestive juices. Dr. Norman Walker's books are listed in the back.

When starches, grains and sugars (generally referred to as carbohydrates) are eaten during the same meal in which any protein is included, we have a serious chemical situation to contend with. This is how it works. The digestion of carbohydrates is interfered with by the presence of the acid material and at the same time the digestion of the proteins remains incomplete in the presence of the alkaline digestive juices. The result is the fermentation of the carbohydrate and the putrefaction of the protein foods. This is not a theory, not a fantasy. This is basic science. The results are very real. They have been proven far too often to leave any room for doubt in the minds of any but those who love their meat and potatoes so much they're blind to the facts.

The idea of eating cooked food is very normal practice today. We are suffering from diseases caused by such foods. Until we decide to go back to Nature we will continue to suffer from degenerative disease. Billions of dollars are spent on treating the symptoms not of our true cause (cooked food) in vain. Please think about this now. Search, explore the truth and you will be free of disease forever. Truth is simple, so simple we have a tendency to overlook it.

The Healing Process:
Understanding Regeneration Reactions

When an individual begins a new health regimen using a cleansing dietary program and/or an alternative therapeutic process, there are always many beneficial systemic and metabolic changes that begin to take place.

Most individuals, occasionally during the elimination and healing process, will periodically experience uncomfortable symptoms along with periodic cycles of feeling much stronger, more energetic, a sense of well-being and clearer, calmer mental and emotional processes. The stronger, healthier, more positive cycles will become more consistent, more the norm with time.

Some of the most common uncomfortable symptoms some individuals report are intermittent and temporary reduction of energy; this is caused by occasional high demand for energy internally to assist the body in its efforts to eliminate residual toxins and poisons from the system, as well as to assist the body in the healing and regeneration of tissues. A simple analogy or comparison to this process takes place when we eat a large meal. When this happens most people feel increased tiredness and are less inclined to mental or physical activity. This occurs due to a substantial amount of the body's nerve energy being temporarily and partially withdrawn from the brain and central nervous system. At the same time a substantial portion of the body's blood supply is temporarily withdrawn from the muscles in order to focus on the vital internal requirement of digestion and assimilation of nutrients consumed during the meal. Therefore we experience less energy externally due to the high demand for energy internally to facilitate the vital requirements of digestion and assimilation. When the digestive process nears completion, the nerve energy and blood supply are once again released for mental and physical activity, our energy returns more fully and we are more capable, and inclined to mental and physical activity once again.

This digestive process and its temporary internal demand for energy is very similar to the internal demand for the body energy internally when we are experiencing elimination and healing reactions. These internal elimination and healing reactions are at a much deeper level internally and more profound in Nature. Therefore, these cycles of elimination and healing require more substantial internalization of energy; thus temporary, periodic external fatigue periods are longer lasting than a simple digestive process and may go on for a period of days or weeks.

It is very common for some individuals to require more sleep, feel like napping in the afternoon, or feel fatigue upon waking in the morning as every cell and tissue, every gland and organ focuses its energy internally to eliminate and heal especially during the sleep process.

Other common reactions some individuals report are aches and pains in various parts of the body. These aches and pains are caused by the catabolic or breakdown of once-virulent, chronic infections. toxic substances and consequent drawing and removal of those toxins from the glands, organs, cells and tissues. This relatively inert toxic material can periodically congest the blood and lymphatic systems. This process then occasionally puts pressure on surrounding tissue and nerves which can cause mild temporary discomfort or pain.

Also, the elimination of acid-based toxins themselves can cause a temporary uncomfortable or painful reaction in the system. Some individuals experience temporary occasional digestive system distress such as gas, constipation, diarrhea, bloating, nausea, headaches, or other digestive system related complaints. The reason for this is the intestines are one of the largest systems of elimination we have. Periodically the liver will release high levels of toxic material it has filtered out of the blood and release these toxins into the duodenum and into the intestinal tract. Also the blood and lymphatic system will periodically release high levels of toxins directly into the intestines for final elimination. There will also be a breakdown and release of old impactions from the large intestine for final elimination. All or any of these processes can cause temporary digestive distress, nausea, headaches, etc.

Other individuals may experience substantial discharge of residual toxins from the mucous membrane linings in the body. These residual toxins may periodically and intermittently be conveyed to the "internal external" areas of the body, the mucous membrane linings, for final elimination.

Western medicine over the last many years has identified some eighty to two hundred viruses that cause the common cold. These viruses have been noted in extensive studies over many years with thousands of cold sufferers. Five thousand years of Oriental medical history and practice states colds and flu are a positive and healthy elimination process of the body in which viruses can participate. In fact these viruses do not cause the cold or flu but they can and do exacerbate, aggravate and perhaps even initiate cold and flu elimination processes.

If the individual has had an accumulation of old infections or toxic residual materials in or around the sinus, upper respiratory system, bronchial passages, lungs, etc., the body will often use these systems to facilitate the clearing and cleansing of the old residual toxins through these areas for final release. When this happens individuals may experience slight clear post-nasal drip, stronger sinus drainage, substantial cold or flu symptoms, or coughing. This helps to bring toxins to the mucous lining surface and then discharge them completely. Sneezing performs a similar function to the cough in discharging mucous, phlegm and other toxins out of the body. Some individuals may experience excessive tearing from the eyes that can cause temporary itching or crusting. Itching and excessive drainage involving the eyes can occur due to strong liver elimination and drainage from the ear due to substantial kidney elimination.

Sometimes there can be temporary, periodic swelling of the throat or tonsils due to congestion of toxins in preparation for final elimination.

Occasionally the body may release residual toxins from the body's lower mucous membrane linings, such as the bowel, bladder/urethra, or the vaginal tract (which might appear to be a bowel, genitourinary, or vaginal yeast infection). This may occur if there has been an accumulation of old infectious or toxic temporarily heavier, irregular, or intermittent menstrual periods or spotting. These discharges may create urinary or vaginal burning or discomfort as acid-based toxins are released from the body.

Occasionally individuals will experience periodic temporary skin reactions such as a rash, pimples, blisters, swelling, itchiness, etc. The reason behind this is quite clear. The skin is the largest elimination system of the human body and there is a direct correlation between the kidneys and the skin that Oriental medicine refers to as the third kidney. One of the primary functions of the kidneys is to filter acid-based toxins out of the blood. When the kidneys are not capable of functioning at optimum levels due to chronic low or moderate levels of infection, inflammation or toxicity, they are not able to filter the blood properly. Also when there is a temporary periodic release of acid-based toxins into the blood as a result of the elimination process, a brief, temporary overload is created as the present weakened capability of the kidneys is unable to filter these toxins adequately. The excess residual toxins, due to temporarily inadequate kidney capability, are deposited back into the blood stream. The blood then takes these toxins to the third kidney - the largest system of elimination we have, the skin.

This is the origin of all skin problems and diseases that can be aggravated or exacerbated by infections. Nothing will manifest on the surface of the skin that is not caused by a "massive discharge of toxins from the kidneys."

The healing and the elimination processes in relation to the blood will periodically and often dramatically alter the blood chemistry profiles. This is due to the healing processes (as the body concentrates blood constituents at the cellular level) and the elimination processes (as the body periodically discharges substantial amounts of residual toxins from the cells into the blood for final elimination). These are two examples of how the regeneration and elimination processes alter the blood chemistry profile. The blood chemistry profile includes some of the following: sedimentation rates, erythrocyte levels, leukocyte levels, acid and uric acid levels, red blood cells and other microscopic blood evaluation visuals. They can often be temporarily skewed and unreliable in terms of orthodox blood profile evaluations.

These symptoms occur because the body is simultaneously

or intermittently healing and eliminating, discharging and ridding itself of residual substances and dead, inert cellular debris from once-virulent infections or toxins that were creating the symptomatic ill health and disease process that were accumulating within the body and interfering with optimum functioning.

As these substances - these neutralized, once-virulent infectious and toxic substances - are ejected from the tissues, they are deposited into the system for final elimination. This temporarily makes the body more uncomfortable until the toxins can be fully excreted.

The body will not generate a fever if there did not exist the internal need to burn off excess animal proteins and fats. Fevers have tremendous therapeutic benefit and should not be stopped or reduced artificially.

Just as an infected wound on the surface of the body will never heal until it is fully cleansed, similarly these infectious and toxic areas in the body, often deeply imbedded in the cells, tissues, glands and organs, will not heal and regenerate unless they are fully cleansed. If not detoxified, these conditions will continue to progressively worsen and contribute to more serious disease processes as time goes by.

All ill health conditions, all disease processes are progressive in Nature. This is evident as people age. The reason is profound yet very simple. All infections, toxins, poisons, chemicals, drugs, and environmental pollutants are, to a great extent, cumulative. It is this cumulative process that creates the progressive development of ill health and diseases at all levels from the most mild to terminal. Chronic levels of infection and toxicity are the primary cause of progressive degenerative disease processes and the so-called free radicals, impaired oxygen levels, and premature aging process.

When we become aware of the possibility of progressive degenerative disease processes due usually to weakening health or disease, hopefully we will make every possible effort to assist our body in its healing and regeneration. Drugs, chemicals, pains killers, etc. retard the elimination and healing process, and are best avoided in all but the most extreme conditions. The more serious, the more chronic the health condition, the stronger will be the elimination and healing reaction and the longer it will take to obtain optimum levels of health. The weaker, or slower the metabolic function capability, the more time will be required.

Occasionally old symptoms will recur; old emotions will surface for final release. Let all of these go.

Every human being has had a lifetime (and more, as we are all born with some degree of infection and toxicity during fetal development) to accumulate infections, toxins, poisons, chemicals and environmental toxic materials in our systems. All of these permeate the body tissues, especially the tissues of high fat content like the brain and central nervous system, cardiovascular system, the lungs, liver, gall bladder, spleen, pancreas, intestines, kidneys, bladder, reproductive system, lymphatic system, as well as the glands and other organs, tissues and cells.

The human body has incredible healing and regenerative ability given the opportunity. The blood plasma regenerates in approximately ten days, the white blood cells in twenty to eighty days, most soft tissues regenerate in approximately ninety days, and the red blood cells regenerate in one hundred twenty days. Every cell and tissue in the body, even the oldest, regenerates every seven years. But if there is chronic infection and toxicity in the tissues, they remain - regenerating, producing more and more endotoxins, inflammation, etc., damaging cells and tissues, glands and organs. The more thoroughly and deeply we clean the system, the greater and stronger, more enduring and optimal will be the results.

The more organic and raw the food we eat, the better the quality and integrity of our blood. The better the quality and integrity of our blood, the more effective the elimination and healing processes of the body. This results in a stronger rebuilding of every cell and tissue we regenerate.

If we are fortunate enough to come across and take full advantage of a dietary program that can prevent, reduce and/or eliminate these symptomatic health problems, these often very problematic, serious or even critical levels of infection and toxic conditions the body has accumulated over a lifetime and more, we are greatly benefited. The results, the effectiveness will serve us immeasurably for the remainder of our lives. The elimination and healing processes required will be easily worth the journey.

In today's modern world of highly chemicalized and polluted soil, food products, air, water, and environment, as well as the pressure and stress of daily life, a pure, organically grown form of nutritional supplementation is extremely important, if not an absolute necessity. Living food is a foundation of life and life is a manifestation of living food.

The soil in which our fruits and vegetables are grown and fruits and vegetables themselves are permeated, genetically altered, sprayed, processed and often coated with toxic chemicals. These chemical fertilizers, pesticides, insecticides and waste contaminates enter the food chain and are in almost everything we eat. These toxic chemicals invariably end up in continually accumulating amounts in our bodies.

The animals from which we obtain a large portion of our foods are continuously fed antibiotics, hormones, steroids, and other chemicals to supposedly prevent infections, promote growth and increase weight for maximum market return. The feed these animals consume also has high concentrations of drugs and toxic chemicals which end up in our bodies in ever-increasing and accumulating amounts, subtly and often severely affecting our health, depressing our immune systems, adding toxicity and proven carcinogenic substances. Now here is a reason not to eat domesticated meat.

Many of the fruits and vegetables we buy at the local market or health food store have been harvested unripe and then often ripened with gas. This immature produce is often stored and shipped over a period of many days, losing whatever nutritional food value it once contained. Your weeds, unless you've sprayed them too, have more nutritional value. Water these weeds, and eat them raw. They have powerful healing effects, mix them with salads.

As a result of the tremendous use of chemicals, processing, storing, transporting and other handling, all of our food products today are severely deficient in the essential vitamins, minerals, trace minerals, amino acids, enzymes and nutrients so necessary for our health and well-being.

With all of this in mind, it should be obvious that there is a tremendous need for pure nutritional whole food in its original form. Buy organic fruits and vegetables, or better yet, grow your own organic garden if you can! The more people who buy organic produce, the cheaper the price will be (supply and demand) for all of us.

We have to give Nature what assistance is possible in the way of removal of the visible handicaps to her work. All disease is ONE THING and subject to the same rules and requiring the same form of treatment. Chemical imbalances of the body have to be corrected through the body chemistry and proper drainage. Stop creating accumulations of acidity the body wants to get rid of - unload the debris of toxins and in the form that it can be eliminated. Do not get in its way with drugs, removal of any organs or blocking a fever. Look to the cause that could be deeply rooted. The cure is always in it. The body accumulates the toxins to the point of tolerance and then it tries to unload them by means of fever, during which the waste is burnt or liquefied and then thrown out. Hyper-acid state of the body is always the cause. Keep it alkaline with organic, raw, fresh fruits and vegetables.

I was helping a man cleanse his body with proper food and juices. He had serious health problems that required thorough cleaning. He went on a twenty-five day juice fast, followed by a water fast of thirty days. On the thirty-first day, he called and said he was having trouble seeing. Whenever he put his glasses on, he would get dizzy, and everything looked blurry. I recommended he get his eyes checked. When he went to an ophthalmologist, the doctor was shocked the man's vision was sixty-five percent better than his prescription indicated. The doctor thought the man had had the wrong prescription all this time. When it was disclosed this man had worn the same glasses for ten years, the doctor simply didn't know what to say. He suggested a brain scan and new glasses. When asked what he thought could have caused the drastic change, the doctor said he had no idea (a miracle).

We knew what it was. The body, after cleansing the debris for about three months, was finally able to absorb the nutrients the eyes needed. Is that simple, or what? You can do the same thing with any of your organs. Just do it wisely and gradually. Ask for help from a true nutritionist or a good naturopathic doctor who knows the laws of Nature. Educate yourself, search, ask questions and look for the real cause of your problems, not just the symptoms. Whatever it is whether it is a toothache or appendicitis, gall bladder or liver, it's still one body.

"All symptoms of all so-called diseases have one origin. All diseases are one. Unity in all things in Nature's plan. Polytheism is gone and everything pertaining to it and coming out of it must go."

J. H. Tilden, MD

Life as it is lived causes the people generally to be enervated. When nerve energy drops below normal, the elimination of toxin (a natural product of metabolism) is checked and it is retained in the blood, bringing toxemia. Toxemia is the first, last and only efficient cause of all so-called diseases.

By now you can clearly see that naming the disease is not going to fix anything. It has to be a whole system, simultaneously or the problem will not be resolved. So whether we like it or not we have to stop doing and putting wrong stuff in our bodies and mind in order to regenerate and heal.

Iridology

"Sit down before a fact as a little child, be prepared to give up every preconceived notion, follow humbly wherever and to whatever abysses nature leads, or you shall learn nothing."
Thomas Huxley

Iridology is a science that involves the use of the iris of the eye to monitor tissue changes that are occurring or have already occurred in the body. It reveals body constitution, inherent weaknesses, strengths, levels of health, and transition that take place in the body due to lifestyle.

Iridology is a system that can scan your whole body without the potentially harmful effects of radiation, chemicals, painful procedures, or excessive expense. It can give you an extremely accurate readout of exactly what is going on in your body now and in the past and your genetic strengths and weaknesses. Iridology can accurately pinpoint the cause of illness to give direction to appropriate methods of treatment. As a result, iridology is used in combination with natural healing methods to prevent illness/disease. I like the way Dr. Michael McCammon, ND puts it: "The iris of the human eye is similar to a computer screen as it displays information on what is held in the database. All it requires is an operator (Iridologist) with the right knowledge and skills to access and interpret the data." The path to optimum health and wellness is shown in your eyes.

Iridology has been practiced for centuries by Native Americans, Ayurvedic physicians of India, the ancient Chaldeans, and many others including our cave-dwelling ancestors who painted irises on cave walls. Its practice fell into obscurity until a Hungarian doctor, Dr. Ignatz von Peczely (1826-1911) rediscovered the art and Iridology found its place in the modern Western world. Today Iridology is a widespread science practiced in many countries of the world including China, Russia, Europe, Australia, New Zealand and the United States. Dr. Bernard Jensen is it's most famous practitioner in the United States and his charts are used worldwide.

How does Iridology work?

In the developing embryo the eye grows out as an extension of the forebrain. Developing as a specialized organ of sight, the eye remains a part of the brain. The iris receives impulses from the entire body giving an up-to-the-minute account of prevailing conditions. The human eye is formed within six weeks of fetal life and is connected via the optic cord. There hundreds of thousands of nerve fibers in the iris and when viewed under an electron microscope, each fiber separates into many more fibers much like an electric cable. All these cables eventually run to the brain, so the iris fibers are very much reflective of brain tissue. The brain is in contact with all the nerves and cells of the body and the iris becomes a screen on which the central and autonomic nervous systems project information about what is happening all over the body at all times.

The iris is like a multidimensional, multicolored holographic display of interpretive data relevant to the health of every individual. **Iridology does not diagnose specific disease**. Iridology plays a role as a *diagnostic* tool in order to clearly demonstrate what happens when disease is suppressed and shows the various levels of information of disease as it progresses. Acute disease shows up as a bright white mark in the fibers of the iris and is associated with pain and inflammation. Sub-acute disease (the beginning of suppression) is displayed as a light gray mark. Chronic disease shows up as a dark gray mark and degenerative disease as a black mark. Remarkably as the body heals, these **signs also change accordingly**, the overall effect being a brightening of the eye. With this analysis, the iridologist can monitor a person's current condition and their progress toward health and wellness.

The observations gained from much time and expense gathering empirical data have made this the most accurate map of the iris available. It is used by iridologists the world over, a testimony to its reliability.

Figure 2

CHART TO IRIDOLOGY

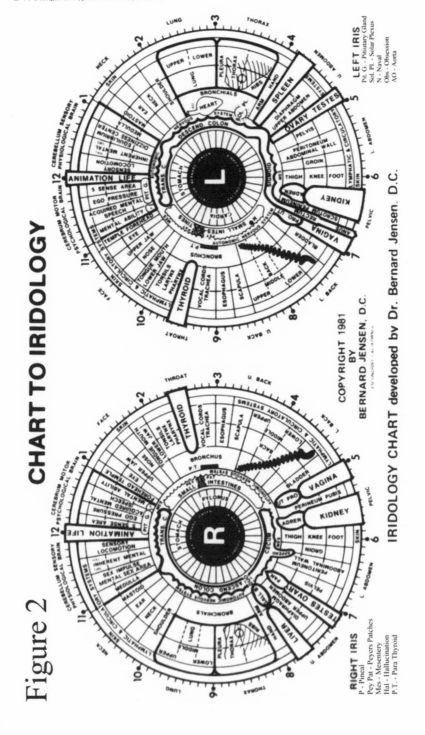

COPYRIGHT 1981
BY
BERNARD JENSEN, D.C.

IRIDOLOGY CHART developed by Dr. Bernard Jensen. D.C.

LEFT IRIS
Pit. G. - Pituitary Gland
Sol. Pl. - Solar Plexus
N - Naval
Obs - Obsession
AO - Aorta

RIGHT IRIS
P - Pineal
Pey Pat - Peyers Patches
Mes - Mesentery
Hal - Hallucination
P.T. - Para Thyroid

Dr. Bernard Jensen s Iris Charts:
Figure 3

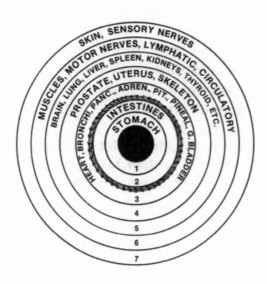

THE IRIS IS DIVIDED INTO 7 ZONES.

Figure 4

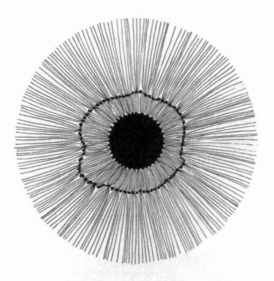

THE AUTONOMIC NERVE WREATH IS
A MAJOR LANDMARK.

The iris map is designed to make this science understandable. The left iris corresponds to the left side of the body and the right iris, to the right side. The iris is mapped into zones radiating from the center outward.

Zone 1:	Stomach
Zone 2:	Small intestine and bowel
Zone 3:	Heart, pancreas, pituitary gland, adrenal glands, gall bladder, solar plexus, parathyroid, bronchioles, bronchus, uterus and prostrate.
Zone 4:	Lungs, ribs, liver, pelvis, brain, kidney, bladder, ovaries.
Zone 5:	Esophagus and spleen.
Zone 6:	Arteries, lymph nodes, muscles and veins.
Zone 7:	Skin and sensory nerves.

These are further divided into sections as a clock face for ease of location, and by cross-matching, the iridologist can identify and describe each location. For instance, the heart is in the left iris at 3:00, Zone 3. The iris signs give indications of function or dysfunction, metabolic waste settlement and vitamin or mineral deficiencies, etc.

The map is like a wheel, the digestive system being the hub. We know that embryonic organs, glands, and tissue develop first from the gut of the growing fetus. All organs and tissues continue to be dependent upon the gut for nourishment and therefore a reflex relationship to these areas exists (as seen in Zone 1 and 2 of the map). The organs are the hub of the wheel and the glands and tissues are the spokes. Like on a bicycle wheel, the hub is the most essential part. The wheel can still function with a few missing spokes, but cannot do without the hub.

Iridology clearly demonstrates it is the digestive systems of the stomach and bowel, then the pancreas and liver that need to be taken care of first. **Every cell of the body is dependent on a healthy digestive and elimination system**. We cannot treat the symptoms without finding the cause.

Iridology is a science whose time has come. Modern medical technology has reached a point where it cannot see the forest for the trees.

In an age of CAT or PET scans, MRI, and ultra-sound analysis, something is fishy when a person can go to six different health practitioners and get half-a-dozen diagnoses. That something fishy is that our approach to medical assessment has been specialized to such a degree we have lost sight of the whole person as they are progressing or declining in health. The unfortunate result of this is rampant levels of misdiagnosis, ill-designed treatment programs, misuse of antibiotics, unnecessary surgery, and widespread medication abuse.

A practical, effective solution to this problem of overall health assessment is the science of Iridology. The iris of the eye reveals body constitution, inherent weaknesses, levels of health and the transitions that take place in a person's body as they interact with their environment. With this map in hand, decoding a person's overall health status, the health practitioner can easily move in the direction most beneficial to the client, in addition to gauging how well the body is healing itself and at what rate. It also shows if the doctor is helping with the right treatment for you.

Many primary care physicians have used this form of analysis to facilitate a more complete understanding of their patients' health care needs.

The eyes have been proclaimed throughout the ages as the windows of the soul. We acknowledge them as the mirror of the body and a person's state of health.

Reflexology

Reflexology is both old and new. Its origins may be traced back to the Chinese who some 5,000 years ago practiced a form of treatment using pressure points. Other ancient cultures in Japan, India and Egypt worked on the feet to promote well-being. Reflexology was being practiced as early as the 6th Dynasty in Egypt (about 2,330 BC). Evidence has been discovered in the tomb of Ankhmahor, also known as the Physician's Tomb. There is evidence, too, that shows Native Americans and tribes in Africa employed some form of Reflexology.

At the beginning of the 20th century, Dr. William Fitzgerald systematized the body into zones. The treatment that emerged from his research was later known as Zone Therapy. One of the students of Zone Therapy was Eunice Ingham, a Physiotherapist. She argued that since the zones ran through the entire body, it would make sense to target the feet for treatments, as they were more accessible and very sensitive. Eunice Ingham should be credited with being the first person to separate the practice of working foot reflex areas from Zone Therapy in general. She charted the body onto the feet, and thus the maps for modern Reflexology evolved.

The goal of Reflexology is the restoration of a state of balance. If the person is to be healthy, all systems of the body must work together in harmony. If any part is out of alignment, other parts suffer as a consequence. The feet have a special relationship with the body. There are 7,200 nerve endings present in the feet that interconnect with every part of the body. By applying a specific pressure massage it is possible to trigger the body to correct imbalances, to stimulate or calm underactive or overactive areas respectively, to cleanse and revitalize that stagnated area and bring in the healing.

Based on the theory the body is divided into 10 longitudinal zones: five on each side of a meridian line through the body. Each zone relates to one of the digits on each side of the body:

1) Zone One extends from the thumb up the arm to the brain and then down to the big toe.

2) Zone Two extends from the second finger up the arm to the brain and then down to the second toe.

3) Zones Three, Four, and Five similarly extend from the remaining third, fourth, and fifth fingers up the arm to the brain and down to the corresponding toes on each side of the body.

Figure 5

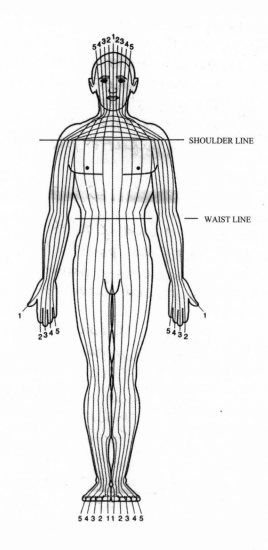

These longitudinal zones are of equal width and extend right through the body from front to back. All organs and body parts lie along one or more of these zones. Working any zone in the foot affects the entire zone throughout the body.

In addition to these ten zones, there exist in the body three transverse zones: across the shoulder girdle, across the waist, and across the pelvic floor. These areas can be transposed onto the feet. The longitudinal and transverse zones together form a grid within which the reflex areas can be located.

Reflex areas corresponding to all the parts of the body are also found in the hands. They are very similarly arranged to those in the feet, but as the hands are smaller than the feet, reflex areas here are correspondingly smaller and a little more difficult to determine precisely. They also tend to be less sensitive due to the constant use of the hands. However in cases where treatment of a foot or both feet is not possible because of injury or infection, the hands may be treated instead.

The thumb is used to apply pressure to the reflex area. The thumb, right or left, is held bent, and the side and end of the thumb are pressed firmly onto each reflex point. The therapist's hands carry out complimentary function during treatment: one working and pressing, the other supporting.

Reflexology is a holistic therapy and seems to treat not only symptoms but also the causes of symptoms. It activates the self-healing mechanisms of the body. Improvement is brought about after one or two sessions if it's not a chronic complaint. Those take longer to correct. Factors such as diet, lifestyle and outlook play a big part in the healing process. Once you become more responsible for your own health, the body will respond more rapidly to healing.

I use Reflexology as a diagnostic tool. It balances the energy flow and eliminates potential problems in their early stages. Pain occurs in areas where energy blockages are present. It's very relaxing and the whole body feels comforted and reassured, calm, energized, and rejuvenated.

Blood System

The human body contains only five quarts of blood. Four quarts fill the blood vessels and are constantly circulated. The blood is composed of microscopic blood cells, approximately twenty-five billion in an average healthy individual. The blood cells travel very fast throughout the body, to carry oxygen and other nutrients to supply the body and the heart.

Every second of the day and night more than two billion blood cells travel to the breathing chambers of the lungs to get rid of waste from the body in the form of molecules, or carbonic acid gas, in exchange for atoms of pure oxygen. You must appreciate this fact in order to keep the blood stream at its maximum point of efficiency so that you can be healthy.

Every blood cell carries food, oxygen and debris. We have to stay pure in order to help the blood do its job twenty-four hours a day, seven days a week. You blood cells are literally your faithful servants. Do not punish them but rather nourish them and give them the opportunity to cleanse and stay clean.

Toxin is a by-product as constant and necessary as life itself. When the organism is normal, it is produced and eliminated as fast as produced. From the point of production to the point of elimination it is carried by blood; hence, at no time is the organism free from toxin in the blood. In a normal amount, it is gently stimulating; but when the organism is enervated, elimination is checked. Then the amount retained becomes over-stimulating, toxic, ranging from a slight excess to an amount so profound as to overwhelm life.

Every so-called disease is a crisis of toxemia; which means that toxins have accumulated in the blood above the tolerance point, and crisis, the so-called disease (cold, flu, pneumonia, cancer, etc.) is through vicarious elimination. Nature is trying to rid the body of toxins. Any treatment that obstructs this effort of elimination stops Nature in her effort at self-healing. Drugs, feeding, fear and overworking prevent elimination. It drives cold, flu, etc. deeper into the tissue and chronic catarrh forms. Most people are so saturated with the idea that disease must be fought and are not satisfied with natural treatment.

When people demand education-truth, not medication, vaccination and immunization, they will get it.

Eat raw fruits and vegetables so you can have clean, non-sticky blood. Eat weeds like dandelion leaves or flowers. Yes, those same plants you try so hard to get rid of in your lawn!

Read more on this subject and the real truth about our chemistry and biology in Dr. Norman Walker's book in the recommended reading section.

The following chart is from Mildred Carter's book **Healing at Your Fingertips:**

Figure 6

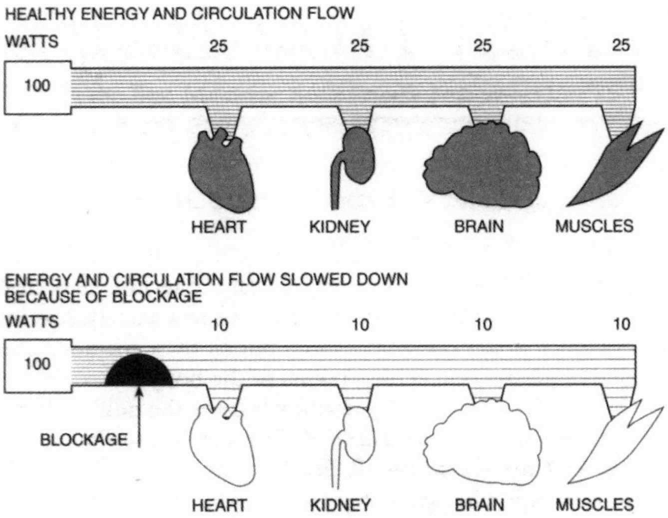

HEALTHY ENERGY AND CIRCULATION FLOW

WATTS 25 25 25 25

100

HEART KIDNEY BRAIN MUSCLES

ENERGY AND CIRCULATION FLOW SLOWED DOWN BECAUSE OF BLOCKAGE

WATTS 10 10 10 10

100

BLOCKAGE

HEART KIDNEY BRAIN MUSCLES

The Lymph System

If all the lymph vessels in the body were placed end to end in a straight line they could cover a distance exceeding 100,000 miles. Their job is immense. The walls of the intestines are filled with lymph nodes or knots which guard the passages into the body against intrusion by destructive substances and fluids. Millions more are located at strategic points throughout the body.

Lymph is formed from fluid, electrolytes and protein that filters through the arterial ends of the enormous number of capillaries. The lymph carrying tissue waste products re-enters the capillaries at their venous ends by virtue of differences in blood pressure, osmotic pressure and intercellular pressure. Lymph vessels and nodes make up a lesser-known system which carries fluid back to the nervous system.

The lymph nodes are located throughout the body as connectors of sorts, where tissue-draining lymph vessels join to the lymph trunks leading back to re-enter the venous system via the subclavian vein. It is in these modes that lymphocytes (a type of white blood cell) are made. The lymphocyte has the ability to pass through vessel and cell walls and to engulf foreign material and organisms that invade the body; so we can see the importance of a healthy lymphatic system in both functions of lymphocyte formation and in moving waste and invaders from body tissue.

The lymphatic system is one of the basic systems that affect everything in the body. It affects the defense and homeostatic systems because, in the case of the defense system, it is part of the immune system and with homeostasis it helps maintain the correct environment for all cells to thrive.

A special refined quality of lymph known as cerebrospinal fluid cushions the brain and spinal cord against the walls of bone that protect them. The condition of this lymph is of the greatest importance in the mental and physical well being of the individual. It is renewed, exchanged and absorbed, as the need arises, by the tiniest, finest, microscopic capillaries of the brain's blood vessels.

The brain and spinal cord are of such extreme importance that simple things like standing up, walking, running or any movement are entirely dependent on their balanced relationship and healthy functioning. The muscles receive their impulses for these activities from the spinal cord while their coordination emanates from the brain.

Lymph is the most important element in maintaining physical balance. The ear channels are filled with lymph and their level changes as we move our head one way or another. The changing of the level causes a greater or lesser pressure on the sensitive nerves connected with the walls of the lymph chambers which in turn send impulses to the brain and spinal column enabling us to maintain equilibrium.

Now you can see how essential it is to keep the microscopic lymph and blood vessels clean and clear of impactions and debris. Only by doing so can the body retain its resilience, buoyancy, youthfulness and health. Don't plug any of these capillaries and destroy their function.

Anything that is not natural will clog them up and cause problems like: soft tissue pain, fibrocystic disease, PMS, inflammation, intestinal syndromes, diabetes, arthritis, bursitis, swelling, bruising and edema.

Now you know how you can get better! You can do this by eating live foods that are mucous free and energy giving to every cell of the body. Cleansing, nourishing and self-discipline are the keys. They are the only true means. We are responsible to keep the blood clean and pure. Nobody can help us with any drugs or surgery if we don't look to the cause. The last fifty years of our evolution we have strayed away from Nature more than the total millions of years and it's showing and surfacing. The consequences are here.

See also Chapter Four: **Alternative Treatments and Lymphatic Drainage Massage.**

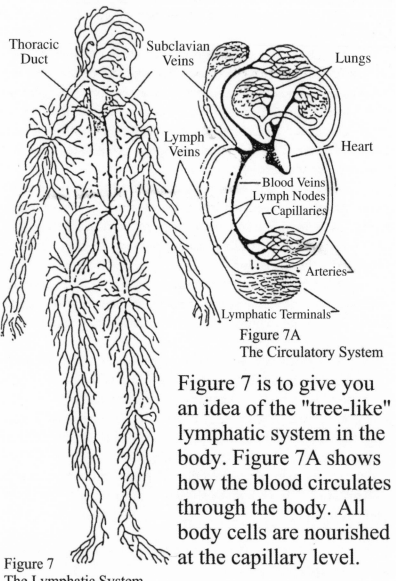

Thoracic
Duct

Subclavian
Veins

Lungs

Lymph
Veins

Heart

Blood Veins
Lymph Nodes
Capillaries

Arteries

Lymphatic Terminals

Figure 7A
The Circulatory System

Figure 7
The Lymphatic System

Figure 7 is to give you
an idea of the "tree-like"
lymphatic system in the
body. Figure 7A shows
how the blood circulates
through the body. All
body cells are nourished
at the capillary level.

Herbs

And God said, "Behold, I have given you every herb-bearing seed, which is upon the face of all the earth, and every tree, in the which is the fruit of a tree yielding seed, to you it shall be for meat.

"And to every beast of the earth, and to every fowl of the air, and to every thing that creepeth upon the earth, wherein there is life, I have given every green herb for meat: and it was so."

Genesis 1:29, 30

To fully comprehend the relationship of herbs to food and a more precise definition of herb, it is important to define the relationship of herbs to our everyday vegetables. According to the *Standard Cyclopedia of Horticulture*, a vegetable "is an edible herbaceous plant or part thereof that is commonly used for culinary (kitchen or edible) purposes." Believe it or not, the word *vegetable* came into existence only about three hundred years ago, since at that time all of our everyday vegetables were known as *herbs* - even such commoners as the beet and carrot. And until vegetables came into use as we know them today, many were used as curative medicines (as they still are in herb-based treatments), just as today these very ones so highly recommended by the medical laity as "protective foods" or "preventive medicines" without which the various organs of our body cannot properly function.

We need to remember that all of our familiar vegetables, such as carrots, onions, fruits or berries, were at one time wild plants and are descendants of the wild carrot (Queen Anne's Lace), wild onions, and wild berries. These descendants were "improved" through cultivation and selection. Unfortunately, this is where we first began to stray from Nature's path, and continue to go astray today. Man, with all his technology, cannot improve Nature.

It's very important to eat herbs of all sorts. They have more power and healing elements than any vegetable of today. One reason our immune system is not as strong as it used to be is due to a lack of powerful herbs - plants we no longer eat or use in our everyday diet. Plus we are destroying them through cooking.

Don't be afraid to try some different herbs, fresh or brewed as sun tea. For every problem and weakness we have, there is an herb to help strengthen your body and mind.

It is of most importance to use herbs that are growing wild since they have their true properties left in them. In other words they are in their original form not hybrids or genetically engineered like our domesticated fruits, vegetables and herbs. This is why herbs can save us and strengthen us. We need them today more than ever. It's not always enough just to have organic herbs but to have them wild. They are much more powerful. They have kept us going for millions of years. All the new vegetables of today are worthless if compared to the power of herbs. Herbs heal us and strengthen us. If not for herbs and their wonderful flavors people would never eat processed foods.

There is an herb or many that will help strengthen each part of the body and its function.

They can contribute to supplying needed enzymes for stimulating metabolic functions of various types and supporting the healthy actions of organs and tissues. Plants-herbs can also supply natural chemotherapy agents for stimulating the cleansing of the system when degeneration has created toxic conditions. Some herbs can help direct the body chemistry into a more efficient range of function so the body can heal itself.

Today we will see more and more use of herbs in their original form as we try to return back to Nature and natural healing. I truly believe that herbs will help save us again. Take a look at the next page.

Traditional Chinese Medicine: Herbalism

In western medicine germs and viruses are considered the primary causes of disease. There is no disease without fertile soil and cause.

In Chinese medicine, the causes of disease are divided into three categories:

1) The six external atmospheric energies: wind, dampness, dryness, heat (fire), cold, and summer heat (a combination of heat and damp, or humidity).
2) Internal causes (which include the seven emotions).
3) Fatigue and incorrect foods.

In nature, extreme wind, dampness, dryness, heat and cold can cause chaos in the world. These same forces can upset the balance in the human body, weakening and obstructing it and causing disease.

Wind is in motion and moves constantly, so when a patient is under the attack of wind the symptoms move around the body, change quickly and seldom last long (an example would be a cold). Wind causes shaking symptoms such as dizziness and muscular twitching.

Dampness is heavy and can cause phlegm or edema; it is one of the main pathogens causing eczema.

Dryness causes chapping and cracking, constipation, withered and broken hair and dry coughs.

Fire can be seen as inflamed tissue, skin eruption, ulcers, and yellow-green bloody discharge.

The nature of cold is to contract and freeze, so the affected patient will feel cold. Pain is frozen in one place and discharges are clear.

Summer heat is a combination of heat and damp as seen toward the end of summer; it can manifest as diarrhea and fevers with profuse sweating.

Herbal medicine today uses all the past wealth of information and experience in combination with modern research and knowledge of plants. It is concerned with treating the underlying condition as defined by traditional diagnoses, and rarely causes unwanted side effects. In fact, the herbs enhance the therapeutic effect of western drugs so that the dosage of these harsher modern drugs can be lowered and many of their side effects can be counteracted. This is seen particularly in cancer patients, where the side effects of radiation and chemotherapy are dramatically reduced when Chinese herbal medicine forms part of the treatment.

Each herb is categorized in terms of its nature, taste and the particular organ it enters. For example gold thread, cork tree, and skullcap are all classified as "cold" herbs and for that reason are used to treat "hot" disorders such as infections and inflammatory illnesses including mastitis, hepatitis and enteritis. On the other hand, cinnamon bark and dried ginger are both "hot" herbs and are used to treat "cold" conditions, such as a "cold" arthritis (stiff joints that are cold to the touch and relieved by warmth; the symptoms of "hot" arthritis would be inflamed, swollen, throbbing joints).

Each flavor we taste affects a different organ. For example sour flavors are thought to soothe the liver, while sweet flavors work as a tonic for the spleen. Pungent flavors open up the lungs to clear external pathogens and dry up excess moisture; bitter flavors cool and soothe the heart; salty flavors enter the kidney and soften lumps and nodules.

The taste and therapeutic use of herbs in this way also extends to foods, hence herbal therapy and dietary therapy are prescribed together. If a patient has a hot, inflamed, infected condition, for example, he or she should avoid those foods which would aggravate or worsen symptoms - such as spicy hot foods, fried foods, alcohol, and shellfish. For damp conditions like asthma, eczema, sinusitis or obesity, foods that increase the damp pathogens in the body would have to be avoided, like sweet foods and dairy products.

The herbal formula calls for combinations of between two and fourteen herbs. It's prescribed in either pill, powder or extract form or tincture which is most effective.

Herbal medicine views the body as an organic whole. The outer body and the internal organs are considered to be closely interrelated so the traditional diagnostic method of observing, listening, smelling and palpation. Tongue and pulse are used as "maps" to the inner bodily environment. Different areas on the tongue reflect different organs and their condition.

Chinese herbs can be used in conjunction with other related therapies such as Acupuncture.

Dietary advice is of big importance. The herbs work to change the inner environment of the body, both physically and mentally, and slowly bring along changes and relief.

We are truly designed to eat fresh herbs and nourish our body with a proper balance of nutrients found in fruits, vegetables and many so-called weeds.

Traditional Chinese medicine including herbalism certainly works the best when the person is eating in moderation and consuming more raw foods especially wild herbs and berries.

When people started cooking their food in the beginning they did not eat all cooked food like we do today. Little by little we became more and more "processed" and with that our health deteriorated more. You can see where we are today. Most people hardly ever eat raw herbs and wild berries. We have a lot of work to do to bring more awareness and truth about herbs.

Chinese medicine is a complete medical system that has diagnosed, treated, and prevented illness for over 25 centuries.

There are four basic branches to Chinese medicine: Herbalism, Food Cures, Acupuncture, and Manipulative Therapy. Broadly speaking, Herbalism and Food Cures are part of the system of internal medicine; while Acupuncture and Manipulative Therapy are included in the system of external medicine. The first book on Chinese Healing Arts, the *Nei Ching*, was published in AD 400 and known as the *Emperor's Classics of Internal Medicine*. All knowledge of Chinese medicine stems from this book, though its sources are much, much older.

Chinese herbs can treat disease states. They also have a large role to play in enhancing immunity, general energy levels, and longevity. The medicinal use of Chinese herbal remedies has well stood the test of time; developed and first used many millennia ago, they are effective for many of today's common problems. Treatments are based upon clinical experiences observed over and over again, and are still valid today.

The point is to restore harmony and to balance Yin and Yang, wet and dry, cold and heat, inner and outer, body and mind. This is all achieved by the regulation of Qi (Chi or "Chee") and of moisture and blood in the organ networks. Qi is the vital energy that travels through us and allows us to move, think and work. Moisture is liquid that nurtures and lubricates tissue. Blood is the material foundation out of which we create bones, nerves, skin, muscles and organs. The organ network (liver, heart, spleen, lung, and kidney) regulates moisture, blood and Qi, while also governing certain mental faculties and all physical activities.

The Chinese believe that emotions are connected to these internal organs. Each internal organ is responsible for a specific emotion, and conversely, each emotion acts on a specific internal organ. Thus the heart gives rise to joy, the liver to anger, the lungs to anxiety and sadness, the spleen to worry and thought, and the kidney to fear.

Acupuncture, Yin-Yang

Chinese medicine has a long history. Five thousand years ago Taoism, of which Chinese medicine is a part, was an oral tradition passed from family to family through stories, poems, songs and myths. Around 3,000 years ago the oral traditions were written down becoming the foundation for the *Nei Ching*, the Chinese Healing Arts.

The development of Acupuncture needles began during the Chang Dynasty, 1766-1154 BC. Physicians began to use stone probes to adjust the flow of energy in the body and help their patients maintain harmony in the body, mind and spirit. Acupuncture is one way of establishing this harmony according to and within the Taoist tradition. It is known as one of the "strands of eight brocades". The other seven are: herbal therapy, dietary therapy, heat therapy, Taoist massage, Acupuncture, Tai Qi (or Tai Chi) and Qi Gong.

Since this system of medicine began little has greatly changed. These are the laws of Nature and of the human being's place within these laws.

The reason I love certain aspects of Chinese medicine is because it does not separate a person's health from his or her position in the universe, spiritual aspirations, emotional world, or ability to be independent and self-sufficient. The more we understand ourselves, our connections and the effect we have on our world, the more power and strength we can obtain, and the more fulfilled and loving we will be. We can help ourselves to do this by understanding the underlying philosophy of Chinese medicine.

"The nameless is the beginning of heaven and earth, the named is 10,000 things."

Chinese Proverb

The nameless is Qi (Chi), or spark, or energy that moves in everything and is at the heart of Taoist philosophy. It is part of everything and it organizes itself to become everything. When it becomes water it is wet and flows. When it becomes fire it is hot and rises up. When it is air we breathe it in. It changes in the body and we breathe it out as carbon dioxide. It is all Qi and it changes its form, but remains Qi. Everything is connected by it and when we understand it we can use it positively from within ourselves and our environment. If we are exhausted because Qi is not flowing in the body, we can learn to unblock it, in this case with needles, but diet or exercise or a change in mental attitude can have a similar effect.

The Chinese first described Qi as polarizing into Yin-Yang:

"Under heaven all can see beauty as beauty, only because there is ugliness. All can know good as good only because there is evil. Therefore, having, and not having, arises together. Difficult and ease compliment each other. High and low rest upon each other. Voice and sound harmonize each other. Front and back follow one another."

Once you describe a thing as bound in time you must create its opposite or balance - but these are not static opposites. They also change. Day changes into night, summer into winter, laughter to sadness, fullness to emptiness.

In the body we look at balancing Yin and Yang. When people are Yin deficient they may be hot, over-active, dry, speak rapidly, be sleep-deprived, etc. If the Yang is deficient, there may be slowness of movement, lethargy, sleepiness, poor appetite, and sogginess or wetness in the body.

Acupuncturists can facilitate change by re-balancing the energy. When there is too much cold they warm and where there is too much heat they cool the energy.

After Yin-Yang the Taoists further differentiated everything into five elements or Wu Xu (five moving forces). These are wood, fire, earth, metal, and water. Here again, we see that Chinese medical thinking, as in Taoist philosophy, one thing is not separate from another. Qi is bound only by time and space. So in the human being Qi moves the human, organizes itself into Yin and Yang aspects, and then further branches into Wu Xu.

Nothing is static, there is always a concept of change and growth. Everything is on a continuum. While evaluation is important, judgment is suspended because judgment can cause blockage whereas evaluation allows the process to continue.

"The ten thousand things rise and fall without cease creating yet not possessing, working yet not taking credit. Work is done, then forgotten, therefore it lasts forever."
Nei Ching

Like in Naturopathy and other natural therapies, when a patient comes with an illness, it is seen as part of a whole changing dynamic in their lives, something to direct them in terms of their health and destiny, not something that is static or separate from them. This avoids a lot of over-identification with negative aspects of the self and promotes the patient toward self-responsibility and health.

In this way a patient has a direction to aim for, can learn from the symptoms and their cause, and help regain their health with more control over themselves and the natural world in which they live. Work with, rather than against Nature.

Acupuncture seeks to balance these energies in the body by the use of fine needles placed into specific points. Each point has its own function and its place on a system of meridians or channels. The blocks cause Qi not to flow as it should.

The external causes are when too much cold, heat, damp, wind or dryness invades the system. This occurs usually because the system is already weak.

The internal causes of disease are the five emotions - an excess of joy, worry, grief, fear or anger - that has not been resolved. These influences effect the Qi of the body and have to be freed to continue the flow. With external causes of disease it is necessary for patients to look at nutrition and lifestyle management, with internal, emotional and spiritual management.

Acupuncturists will take your pulse and ask to see your tongue. In traditional Chinese medicine therapists feel the quality of the different pulses under the fingers rather than just the heart rate. Each finger will feel the energy of a particular organ meridian, and how that meridian is functioning in the body.

The tongue is also very important diagnostic tool in traditional Chinese medicine. Sometimes it is even more important than the pulse, as it changes much more slowly and reflects the true inner conditions of the person without responding to different situations (such as stress or exercise) as the pulse does. Western doctors used to check the tongue as part of their normal procedures, but not any longer.

The tongue coating is very important especially in showing the state of the digestive organs. A thick, dry and yellow mucousy coating shows the presence of phlegm - heat in the body that has consumed the Yin fluids. A thick white coating indicates an internal damp, cold condition. There are infinite variations in the tongue and pulse and diagnosing these variations constitutes the skill of the Acupuncturist.

More information on the tongue and location of the organs is included on the pages about Ayervedic medicine.

Qi Gong

The greatest treasure ancient China has bequeathed us is traditional Chinese medicine. It has proven beneficial to the health and longevity of tens of millions of Chinese generation after generation, throughout the ages right down to the present. Now in the West, it is enjoying increasing popularity.

Traditional Chinese medicine is founded on Qi, regarded as the vital force or energy influencing all aspects of health and healing in the mind and body. This vital force can be controlled and strengthened within oneself under the name of Qi Gong along with proper nutrition.

Qi Gong, as a fitness and healing art, has existed for thousands of years, handed down from the mythological realms of time, through ancient times to the modern era. Qi Gong has been synthesized and refined over thousands of years of vast experience, observation, knowledge, research, and practice distilled from many different schools and sources of diverse background. An immense body of literature has developed around this traditional medical art.

Qi Gong is a system ancient in origin of an unfamiliar culture, often mysterious to the West. It's a natural mental and physical exercise that does not engage any religious involvement.

Long known as a simple, gentle, safe, and effective exercise, Qi Gong is used for relaxation, meditation, and physical fitness with small demands on energy, strength, space and time.

Qi has been the fundamental concept in Chinese philosophy regarded as the only elemental substance that possesses force or energy in the universe.

In traditional Chinese medicine, it is believed that life is the result of Qi. To live is to have vital energy-Qi, and to die is to not have Qi. Generally speaking, Qi within the body comes partly from heaven and partly from earth by absorption through lungs, digestive tract and skin. Qi travels the meridians of the body and is stored in the Qi cavities (acupoints) of the meridians, but is not noticed physically. It governs the interplay between Yin and Yang, influences the relationship among the Five Elements, and activates Zang Fu (the internal organs). Every illness can be attributed to the improper function of Qi.

In Chinese, the word Qi (pronounced "Chee") usually means air and respiration but it also has another essential meaning, that of "vital energy" or "life force". In modern scientific terminology the nearest approximation would be "energy" or "power", which enables the machine of the mind/body to work.

The term Gong (pronounced "Kung") has several meanings such as art, skill, work, success, but also exercise, manipulation and self-discipline. A literal translation of the two words together would be "manipulation of vital energy" or "energy exercise".

In the course of a lifetime the mind/body is constantly influenced by every aspect of changing Nature: weather, geographic location, seasons, temperature, colors, foods and emotions. Thus, the circulation of energy needs tuning up periodically, otherwise Qi can become stagnant gradually and then disease occurs. Qi Gong functions as that tuning up.

Qi Gong is an ancient Chinese art in which people are trained to the sensation and manipulation of vital energy by exercising the mind, breath, body or self-massage. With Qi Gong practice a smooth functional activity of the organism and a state of dynamic equilibrium within the body are achieved. Experiencing, balancing, circulating and promotion are the essence of Qi Gong exercise. The goal is to maintain well being in mind and body to prevent disease, to relieve sickness, and to prolong life.

In traditional Chinese medicine exercise should consist of two parts, the inner and the outer, both equally important. The inner exercise influences Jing Luo (meridians) and Zang Fu (the internal organs) while the outer exercise influences the muscles, joints, ligaments and limbs. Qi Gong can accomplish both aspects simultaneously.

Qi Gong is an exercise of preserving and storing body energy. By slowing down the metabolism, the heart rate and respiratory rate are reduced. It is essential, therefore, that above all it be practiced without any undue exertion.

Qi Gong, Tai Ji Quan (known as Tai Chi), and Gong Fu (or Kung Fu, the Chinese martial art) are like triplets. In theory they share many similarities and their training methods overlap.

However, they are different. Qi Gong focuses more on deeper concentration in the mind, the sensation of Qi, and the emission of Qi. By contrast, Tai Ji Quan places more emphasis on body movement with slowness and fluidity, while Gong Fu executes body movement with strength and speed.

In ancient Chinese philosophy Qi can be categorized into three classes: 1) Heaven Qi, consisting of energy from the sun and moon; 2) Earth Qi, from objects like mountains, rivers, plants and living creatures, gravity, and the magnetic field; and 3) Human Qi from within oneself. These three elements integrate and influence each other, resulting in what we, and the surroundings, are today.

The concept of Qi permeated ancient Chinese medical wisdom gradually forming a complex understanding of Qi in the body. The balance and harmony of Qi s the center of human well-being. Different forms of Qi within the body can be classified in accordance with its distribution, source, direction, function, and quality. In addition, various classifications have been made in different schools. To sum up, in medical Qi Gong, there are: 1) Zhen Qi, involved in the function of connecting and nourishing various parts in the body; 2) Yuan Qi, involved in the function of reproduction; 3) Ying Qi, circulating inside the vessels (blood); 4) Da Qi, inhaled and exhaled in normal breathing; 5) Gu Qi, the essence of foods planted on earth. 6) Wei Qi, distributed in muscles, skin, and circulating outside to defend the body against external noxious agents; 7) Xie Qi, elements causing various diseases; and 8) Wai Qi, emitted from some skillful Qi Gong masters.

All the Qi(s) inter-depend, interact, and transform each other.

Chinese internal arts have gained international recognition and warrant scientific research and validation. The practice of Qi Gong is simple to perform by people of any age or ability and is now being made widely available.

Ayurvedic Medicine

Ayurveda defines health as a soundness and balance between body, mind, soul and equilibrium between the *doshas*. According to Ayurvedic medicine, there are seven major factors that can disrupt physiological harmony - genetic, congenital, internal trauma, external trauma, seasonal, natural tendencies or habits, and magnetic/electrical influences. It is believed that disease is the result of a disruption of the spontaneous flow of Nature s intelligence within the human body. When we violate Nature s law and cannot adequately rid ourselves of the results of this disruption then we have disease.

There are pathologies recognized as being genetically based and prompted by environment. Genetically, susceptibility can be triggered in the womb by the mother s lifestyle, diet, habits, activities and emotions. Accordingly individuals possess natural tendencies to adopt certain habits, such as overeating and smoking.

From birth stresses, both inner and outer, challenge an individual s health. Disease can also have an emotional cause such as deep-seated, unresolved anger, fear, anxiety, grief, or sadness. External traumas and injuries can also play an influential role.

Ayurveda also takes into account how the seasons and time of day influence health. Dietary and other therapeutic suggestions are often prescribed with this in mind. Summer s bright light and heat can induce inflammatory conditions such as hives, rash, acne, biliary disorders, diarrhea, or conjunctivitis in susceptible individuals. Autumn reflects windy, dry, cold qualities, which lead to the development of neurological, muscular, and rheumatic problems such as constipation, sciatica, arthritis, and rheumatism. Winter s deep cold and biting wind stresses the respiratory system with colds, hay fever, cough, congestion, sneezing, and sinus disorders. Spring is a combination of winter and summer.

Ayurvedic physicians have traditionally relied on the powers of observation rather than equipment and laboratory testing in diagnosing disease. Diagnosis is based on physical observation, questioning the patient as to personal and family history, palpation (feeling the body) and listening to the heart, lungs, and intestines. This approach is changing however as physicians integrate

Ayurvedic traditions with modern diagnostic methods.

Ayurvedic physicians pay special attention to the pulse, tongue, eyes, and nails. Whereas Western medical doctors use the pulse to determine heart rate, Ayurvedic doctors describe three distinct types of pulses related to the seasons as described above. They can distinguish twelve different radial (wrist) pulses: six on the right wrist, consisting of three deep and three superficial; and similarly six on the left. By focusing on the relationship between the pulses and the internal organs, a skillful practitioner can feel the strength, vitality, and normal physiological tone of specific organs at each of the twelve sites.

Practitioners routinely perform urine examinations to help them diagnose *doshic* imbalance in a patient. An early morning midstream sample of urine is collected and its color observed.

Normal urine has a typical musty smell. A foul odor indicates toxins in the system. A sweet smell indicates a diabetic condition. Gravel in the urine indicates stones in the urinary tract.

The tongue is another diagnostic site. By observing the surface of the tongue and looking for discoloration and/or sensitivity of particular areas, an adept practitioner can gain insight into the functional status of internal organs. For example: a whitish tongue indicates an accumulation of mucus, a dehydrated tongue is symptomatic of a decrease in plasma, while a pale tongue indicates a decrease in red blood cells.

Tongue exams have been used in Chinese, European, and other types of medicine for centuries. Tongues can tell the trained practitioner a lot about a person s health.

Changing a person s diet to more raw fruits and vegetables will change the interior of the body and the tongue will change. Ayervedic medicine pays lots of attention to nutrition. I hope that in the future all of the natural therapies use more living foods to correct any health problems.

Figure 8
Ayervedic Tongue Chart

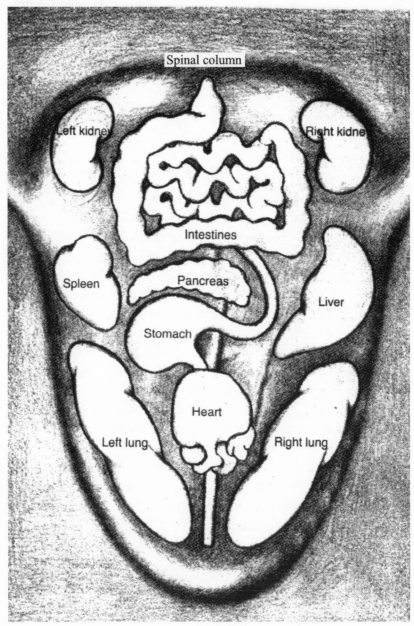

Homeopathy

The man who started Homeopathy was Dr. Samuel Hahnemann, a German doctor, who in 1786 was a very prominent physician and medical author. The form of medical practice at that time did not sit well with him. He wrote:

"I renounced the practice of medicine, that I might no longer incur the risk of doing injury, and I engaged in chemistry exclusively and in literary occupations."

Around the year 1800, while translating the *Materia Medica* (a text concerning the actions and therapeutic effects of substance), by Professor Cullen of London University, Dr. Hahnemann came across a part of the text devoted to the therapeutic indications of Peruvian bark (a source of what is today known as quinine). In *Materia Medica*, Cullen attributed its success in the treatment of malaria to the fact it was bitter-tasting. Dr. Hahnemann found this explanation both vague and irritating to his scientific mind, so much that he did something unusual. He took a series of doses of Peruvian bark himself. It was the action of a man whose approach to medicine was in keeping with this extraordinary experiment. Homeopathy was born.

This was indeed a revelation to Dr. Hahnemann. He had discovered that a drug known to be a curative in cases of malaria actually produced the very symptoms of the condition when taken by a healthy person. This formed the basis of his "Law of Similars" which to this day underpins all Homeopathic thinking.

Homeopathy comes from the Greek *homo(io)*, same, and *pathos*, suffering. The word means to "treat with something that produces an effect similar to the suffering."

Dr. Hahnemann began to have great success in treating illnesses that up until that time had been difficult to manage. Then he moved on to his next discovery. He realized that the actual dosage given to a patient was very important and began to experiment with reducing the dose. He lowered the amount to one-tenth of usual and found the patient was cured, but the aggravation though slighter, remained. He diluted further, each time prescribing one-tenth of the previous dose and finally reached a solution that was ineffective. He came to the belief that if the medicine was not strong enough to aggravate the symptoms, it would be ineffective in bringing about a cure. He found that by strongly shaking the medicine at each dilution, it became not only less toxic but actually more potent and therefore more likely to bring about a cure in the patient. Homeopathy to this day gives substances that are diluted to levels of one part per million and beyond and still bring about a cure in the patient.

He concluded that in every substance in Nature there lay hidden an inner "vital force of life" that could be used to potentiate healing. It was *this* that acted therapeutically, stimulating the person's own vital force or life energy to bring about well being.

"The totality of symptoms is what must be prescribed on, or a remedy found for."

In asserting that the total symptom picture was paramount in matching symptoms to the cause, Dr. Hahnemann was embracing what today is known as the holistic view of illness.

A Homeopath will be interested in all of the patient's symptoms in keeping with the totality of symptoms law. A cure was said by Dr. Hahnemann to be at best "slow, gentle, and permanent."

Dr. Hahnemann not only discovered a new approach to the healing of the sick that he called Homeopathy, but he also gave humanity a method of curing illness from the inside since many times the physical symptoms are the last to disappear. Homeopathy has grown slowly, gently and permanently to every continent and in its time has given back millions of people the health and well being they desperately sought.

Homeopathy will find its true place at the forefront of medicine along with Naturopathy and nutrition in the 21st century.

I remain certain that Homeopathy works the best when a person becomes aware of what they put in their body and follows Nature's laws of cause and effect. Nature heals us if we assist her with natural support.

Herring's Law of Cure states that "all cure comes from within out, from the head down and in the reverse order as the symptoms have appeared in the body" (like our chronic diseases). In changing to the new, we must undergo a reversal process which involves remission of the troubles and illness that exist at the present in the body and which have been experienced in the past. The same path is followed in reverse starting from where you are today so you will relive past problems, recreate past pain and sickness. So if a person has asthma now, he or she will go back into hay fever and finally return to the stage of a cold, bronchial problem, flu and fevers that he or she had in the past. The correction ultimately comes as we go through the retracing steps. Many do not realize that this is the path for regaining health. The body this way cleanses and results in healing crises that are elimination processes initiating the rare occurrence of our old ills and troubles. So do not suppress the symptoms. As Dr. Jensen says "Health is learned and earned."

In the reverse chronological order that the symptoms originally appeared, for example if the patient first experienced kidney pain six years ago, backache eight years ago and a migraine ten years ago, the kidney pain is likely to clear first, then the backache second and the migraine last. For instance, inside the body will heal before the outside can heal.

What you put in your body will determine if it's a healing thing so the body can heal itself. When you have a skin problem you cannot expect to fix it permanently just from the outside by putting cream on it but rather by fixing the inside first, then the outside will also heal. The body also heals from the head down, for instance, the shoulder may heal before the elbow, elbow before the hand, knees before the feet. Your mind has to know what needs to be done in order for it to happen.

By eliminating the causes we can quickly come to most serious releases and cures. As I mentioned earlier good nutrition will help the most, together with other natural therapies.

Absence of Proof is not Proof of Absence

Before rediscovering that the earth was round, people thought that the earth was flat. They would even kill for it. They could not prove that the earth was round. Does that mean that the earth was flat? Did science need to prove that the earth was not flat for the earth to be round? Absence of proof is not proof of absence. Please reflect on this message.

By the time some things are proven many people die in the process. Between the scientific proof and the statistics there is something immense that already is, and that is Nature. She does not need to be proven, she just is. Science pretends to know something that has long been experienced by Nature.

Modern medicine wants proof of something that always was and is and perhaps cannot be proven. Does the proof of absence mean that it is not so? Can science ever make a seed that will grow? Then you might consider science over Nature/God. Until then, keep in mind that nature provides answers when science fails.

Because modern medicine always wants scientific proof we have so many degenerative diseases and problem as never before. We have been tricked and confused. If science does not keep Nature in mind pretty soon there will be no Nature or science left to prove. We simply cannot go against Nature. But with her, we can have a scientific proof of how she works. Only to the point. I have nothing against science. Scientists want to prove how smart they are. While Nature is wise and intelligent and her laws are immutable and that is that. Nothing just happens. Happening is just. We must surrender to Nature-God.

Take a look at how we can help the body cleanse and heal with alternative treatments and with Nature's laws always in mind in order to succeed.

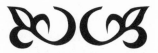

CHAPTER FOUR
Alternative Treatments:
Lymphatic Drainage Massage

It's crucial to mention a very important part of good health and one that helps you get better faster: the lymphatic system.

Lymphatic Drainage Massage is a technique that works specifically on the lymphatic system. Essential oils are combined with massage technique to stimulate lymphatic flow and clear the system of toxins, provided more toxic elements aren't put back into the system.

The lymphatic system carries fluid around the body in a network of branching vessels. The fluid carries nutrients (particularly fat-soluble nutrients) to the tissues and carries fluid and toxins away from the cells. The lymphatic system also plays a part in infection combat and prevention by carrying the body's infection-fighting equipment around the body. There is a link to blood circulation through the lymphatic system via capillaries where tiny vessels of the lymphatic system exchange fluid with equally small blood capillaries. The larger lymphatic vessels connect with the blood stream via the subclavicular veins underneath the collarbone.

The lymphatic system also has collecting points, or nodes, which can be felt as swollen glands under the jaw with infections such as colds or flu. Other nodes are situated in the groin and armpits. There are larger ducts into which tiny tubes of the lymphatic system drain in the abdomen and around the heart. In larger lymphatic ducts lymph fluid is filtered by lymphatic glands. Bacteria and other foreign bodies are collected and lymphocytes produced which help the body fight infection by surrounding and neutralizing invaders. The lymphatic system, unlike the blood circulatory system does not have a central pump and depends on compression from surrounding muscles and general activity of the body to move lymph fluid around.

The efficiency of lymphatic flow is affected by lack of exercise, sedentary work or prolonged spot standing and also clogging with dead, mucousy foods. Massage is used with aroma therapy to stimulate and cleanse the system and consists of a series of treatments generally twice a week over a period of several weeks. LBG (light beam generator) is used to break up congested tissue and improve circulation.

Lymphatic Drainage is very effective in helping boost the immune system. For instance, when the body is prone to recurring infections or when recovering from a bout of illness. Slowly the treatment is combined with strict changes in diet as necessary and an increase in exercise in combination with deep relaxation exercises to balance mind and body and decrease stress levels.

Lymphatic Drainage Massage is very helpful in easing fluid retention in the body and is used extensively in treating the fatty fluid deposits of cellulite. A detoxification diet of raw organic fruits and veggies is also recommended along with a program of exercise, de-stressing techniques, as well as learning about the cause of the person's problem.

Eating organic fruits and vegetables will help thin the blood so debris can move more easily out of the blood and into the lymph system where it gets carried from the body and thus achieves health.

A low-grade infection eats away at healthy tissue and spreads disease everywhere. It is also a main source of irritation tot he entire defense mechanism of the body. Hidden dental infections are huge problems. X-rays can miss things because you cannot see what is in the back of the tooth. Electrical diagnosis of the tooth is far superior but it is not used much in the United States. X-ray may show infection in the tooth going down to a certain depth when in fact it could go much further causing all sorts of health problems. Due to the inflammation a person may feel no pain at all. Before you have any surgery check your teeth first. In many cases they are the biggest culprits.

Dr. Schulze's Intestinal Detoxification Program

Digestive system and colon health have reached an all time low in the United States and worldwide due to the adoption of a more Western life-style that includes eating processed foods. Diseases of the digestive tract are on the rise. The number-one cancer among men and women is colorectal. Modern life has taken its toll on our digestive and elimination organs.

Refined, processed, low-fiber foods; animal fats, lack of exercise, and an increasing level of stress all contribute to our current gastrointestinal health crisis.

The frequency at which a normal healthy person should move their bowels has been a great misconception among the public and medical professionals alike. For years doctors have believed that anywhere between one bowel movement a day and one a week was normal. When we examine more simple cultures we find their bowels move much more frequently, two to three times a day on average. This of course is due to the fact these people eat better and less-processed foods, get more exercise, and have much less stress.

Dr. Schulze has found it is normal to have one bowel movement a day for each meal you eat. In other words if you eat three meals a day, you should have three bowel movements a day.

The *Merck Manual*, the medical industry's standard text for the diagnosis and treatment of disease tells us colon degeneration is on the rise. The incidence of diverticulosis has increased dramatically over the last forty years. It states that in 1950 only ten percent of adults over the age of forty-five had this disease, in 1955 fifteen percent in 1972 thirty percent, and in 1987 almost half. The latest edition states that the incidence "increases rapidly" over age forty and that "every person will have many" if they live long enough. Every American adult will have herniation of the large intestine.

Diverticula are saccular herniations that protrude through the wall of the colon. These "bowel pockets" are almost always asymptomatic (you can't feel them). They are caused by a sluggish, constipated bowel. These pockets fill with old fecal material that can be reabsorbed into the bloodstream. This can infect the entire body causing all types of toxic reactions.

A sluggish bowel can retain pounds of old, toxic and poisonous fecal matter. Many times the real cause behind sickness and disease is retention and re-absorption of this toxic waste.

The first step in everyone's health program should be stimulating, cleaning and toning all the elimination organs and the bowel is the best place to begin.

Watch what you do to your body from now on! Keep the bowel clean and make certain you eat non-processed food. No man-made stuff, only what Nature provided for you and in its original form - raw.

Dr. Schulze's patients have all gotten better, and rid of some of the deadliest diseases by cleansing the bowel and elimination channels. You can do the same.

The first step is to clean out the bowel and make sure it stays working properly. It's easy t do when you eat unprocessed foods. That will keep all other elimination channels working better. Other organs won't have to take up the burden and work harder.

The second step is to keep putting the proper nutrients in your system - raw fruit and vegetables - so the bowel will flush out any toxins better.

Finally comes the support and strengthening of the body so it won't be susceptible to lazy targets like mucous plaque and toxic environment.

Put only the good stuff in. Become aware of what you eat, think, and do. Remember food is the foundation of life and life is a manifestation of food!

For bowel problems, you may contact Dr. Schulze directly at 1-800-HERB-DOC (1-800-437-2362)

Colon Health and Cleansing

We are slowly building up toxic residue from all the high-stress foods and combinations we have been eating over a lifetime. Refined products, sugar, chemicals, additives, preservatives, salt, pasteurized milk products, hydrogenated and rancid fats all lead to toxic buildups in the body and to further fatigue, lack of vitality and disease.

The result of eating a high-stress standard American diet (SAD) from infancy to adulthood leads to a thick mucus buildup throughout the digestive tract preventing proper assimilation of nutrients from the food we eat. A normal healthy colon should eliminate two to three bulky stools each day. Some health authorities even suggest it's best to eliminate after each meal. However the average American diet of too much de-vitalized food clogs the colon and wastes stagnate in it.

Today with modern toilets that are one and a half feet off the ground makes constipation even worse. The lack of squatting down does not push the fecal matter out completely without straining. You can put your feet up higher on a bench or a box and squat down like our ancestors did. Raise your hands above your head so that the transfers colon [*transverse*] can completely empty with ease.

The stagnant colon contains decaying putrefying matter from wrong food choices and wrong food combinations. Scientists have found thirty-six poisons produced as a result of putrefaction from constipation that are absorbed through the walls of the intestines and get into the bloodstream, lymphatic, nervous system, circulatory system, and to the entire body. Along with these poisons can be food colorings, food additives, preservatives, pesticides and other chemicals in and on our food. The liver is the first line of defense to try and keep these poisons from entering the body but because of too many toxins it becomes overloaded and cannot handle this load.

The toxicity arising from the colon is a major cause of degenerative disease. At a seminar in Great Britain attended by leading physicians in the Royal Society of Medicine, it was explained how poisons are constantly bathing delicate body cells and setting up changes which finally result in grave disease.

The British physicians concluded that the colon and subsequent poisoning from it leads to infections, cancers, headaches, leg pains, arthritis, depression, insomnia, chronic fatigue, difficult concentration, wrinkles, boils, eczema, herpes, lupus, acne, female problems, premenstrual syndrome, circulatory, kidney, liver, respiratory, and colon problems. The list of diseases they gave are inclusive of almost all degenerative diseases of today. These diseases all responded favorably when the toxic colon was dealt with and raw fruits and vegetables in every day diet.

A toxic body becomes a sick body. Dr. Norman Walker, who made a lifetime of researching the colon, says it is the number-one affliction underlying nearly every ailment and the primary cause of nearly every disturbance of the human system. The health of the body depends on the colon and toxic buildup in the colon destroys the health.

The elimination of undigested food and other waste products is as important as the proper digestion and assimilation of food says Dr. Walker, in *Colon Health*. Death can be said to begin in the colon. The toxic buildup can interfere with nutrient absorption even when nutritional intake may be adequate. Proteins, vitamins, and enzymes suffer the most. The nutrient absorption can be improved by cleansing the gastrointestinal tract with activated charcoal crystals, psyllium husks, and an herbal laxative. When the colon is first cleansed of old, dehydrated, toxic poisons, a low-stress food-combining diet will have even more of a noticeable and positive impact on one's health.

Few realize that failure to effectively eliminate waste products from the body causes such fermentation and putrefaction that ailments and diseases rapidly proceed. **You will never attain superb health until the old hardened feces within the body are dissolved and removed. In order to become healthy you must have complete removal of old mucoid matter from your colon**.

The most advanced and effective method of cleansing the colon is with activated charcoal crystals (from peach pits and walnut shells), psyllium husks, and a good, gentle, non-habit-forming herbal tablet. Make certain you include fresh fruits and vegetables in your daily diet.

We can make a major impact on the chemicals, additives, high-stress food combinations, and poisons produced from within our colons by cleansing the colon with the charcoal and psyllium. The charcoal has such absorptive powers that it will draw off from the colon walls years of buildup and it will absorb toxins that the body produces from foods that are dead, high-stress, poisonous, or undigested.

The charcoal cleansing program is a powerful way to remove all types of poisons from the bloodstream, liver and colon. It does not interfere with the absorption of nutrients to any significant degree; instead after the waste is removed the assimilation of nutrients will be improved, especially if you continue with a proper diet of raw fruits and vegetables.

The charcoal cleansing program is the most advanced formulation available today for cleansing the colon thoroughly. The results will amaze even the skeptic. One cannot achieve good health unless the system is cleaned out. One must start where the main drain is sluggish or plugged up - the colon. The colon is the main drain and if you could see what has come out of people's unhealthy colons you'd scarcely believe it.

If the colon is sluggish (less than two to three good bowel movements a day, if you eat three or more meals a day), then you cannot have good and vigorous health. If you eat dead, cooked, non-nourishing food, the cells won't be properly nourished, won't regenerate properly, and further disease and breakdown will follow. If the digestive system doesn't work properly, the life-giving cell will be further malnourished and serious disease will manifest itself. The longer these toxins remain in the bowel the more critical the degeneration becomes. It is logical that a person will not improve permanently until the pollution is removed from the system, and a continual diet of good food is supplied to the digestive system and every cell in the body.

The cleansing of the colon can affect many conditions. For example:

Digestive organs: colitis, gastritis, degeneration of the liver,

gas, bloating, diarrhea, constipation, ulcers.

Cardiovascular system: low or high blood pressure,

permanent dilation of the arteries, degeneration of the heart, angina, arteriosclerosis.

<u>Nervous system</u>: headaches, depression, insomnia, chronic fatigue, paralysis.

<u>Eyes</u>: hardening of the lens, cataract, hemorrhage.

<u>Skin</u>: wrinkles, dermatitis, eczema, boils, seborrhea.

<u>Muscles and joints</u>: muscular pain, degeneration of muscles, muscle wasting, breasts, arthritis, rheumatism, urinary tract disease, mastitis.

<u>General disturbances</u>: anemia, lowered resistance to infection, growth retardation, irritability, anger, goiter, tumors, senility, pre-menstrual syndrome, etc.

To cleanse the colon effectively activated charcoal crystals are taken along with psyllium husk and an herbal combination. The cleansing takes at least thirty days and is repeated at least a few times a year. Usually one will rest for a few months and then repeat the cleansing until the person has been feeling well and bowel movements are restored to normal.

Charcoal is a micro-crystalline, non-graphite form of carbon. It is processed from walnut shells and peach seeds. Activated charcoal is the residue from distillation of the organic matter (the shells and pits) that is treated to increase it absorptive power.

Charcoal is processed so that it has a large surface to allow for the maximum absorption of toxins and chemicals within the gastrointestinal tract. It prevents toxins in the colon from getting back into the body. See a health practitioner and follow their advice.

More than anything, continuation of fresh fruits, vegetables and their juices will cleanse, rebuild/restore the body and are recommended to promote and continue good health. It will also continue to strengthen the walls of the bowel as well as other organs. The whole body can be in harmony so that the master gland (pituitary and hypothalamus) can orchestrate and give correct signals to other endocrine system glands (hormone-producing glands) proper messages. This is of most importance and a major cause of our multiple illnesses.

Dr. Richard Anderson - Mucoid Plaque

The phrase, "mucoid plaque", is a term coined by Dr. Richard Anderson, ND, NMD, to describe various conditions found throughout the body, especially in hollow organs and the alimentary canal. It is a substance the body naturally creates under unnatural conditions, such as attack from acids, drugs, heavy metals and toxic chemicals. Mucoid plaque found in the bowel is not equivalent to the natural healthy gastric and intestinal mucus. The natural mucus serves as a necessary buffer of the gastrointestinal wall and as a lubricant for intestinal movement. Mucoid plaque of any description is unnatural and found only after the body has moved toward a diseased state. Medical science has many words to describe each of these conditions but none seem to be an effective term that describes them under one category.

Generally mucoid plaque is composed of mucin, a secretion containing carbohydrate-rich glycoproteins. However there are many other substances that may be involved with mucin, such as lymph, fecal matter, and various types of proteins. Mucins, or glycoproteins, are produced and secreted from salivary glands, the esophagus, stomach, small and large intestine, gall bladder and pancreatic ducts.

Intestinal mucin is designed to protect the intestine under extreme conditions. But abnormal buildups of mucin have been identified with pathogenic bacteria and bowel disease. The main function of mucus is to serve as a protective barrier from acid and enzymes as well as ingested potentially toxic substances (alcohol, aspirin, drugs, sodium chloride, etc.). Mucin is soluble in alkaline water, and is precipitated by acids. In other words acids stimulate mucus secretion when the body is unable to adequately buffer those acids with electrolytes. Stress and eating acid-forming foods drains the body's electrolyte reserves. Therefore, this combination may cause the body to lose its acid buffering efficiency, which contributes toward the stimulation of unnatural mucus secretion.

Natural, normal and healthy mucosa contains large volumes of alkaline buffering agents that protect the bowel wall from invasions of acids and toxins. As long as the proper electrolyte reserves are maintained and nothing has been taken to destroy that important protection we have use of it. However most Americans, and especially carnivorous and milk-drinking Americans, have lost this valuable pH. Not only that but our ingestion of harmful poisons such as drugs, alcohol, sodium chloride, etc., deals consistently hard blows to our digestive protective mechanisms. Unfortunately many doctors are unaware there are two kinds of mucus barriers in the gut. There is the normal intestinal mucus and the pH-mucus barrier. Mucoid plaque overlies the normal mucus.

It is a well-known medical fact that acids induce physiological responses. It has been shown that cancer of the bowel is often associated with bile acids. Mucin and mucus are natural protective liquids that are excreted by the mucous cells, among others, throughout the stomach and intestines to help protect the delicate mucosal membranes from acids and toxins.

Another well-known fact is that 90% of the ulcers that develop in the human body are found in the duodenum (part of the small intestine). This occurs primarily in an area of the duodenum where the Bruner's glands are located. Bruner's glands secrete large amounts of mucus which naturally protect the body from acids. Ulcers develop only after the body has lost its ability to create *alkaline* mucus. The point is acids can severely damage the gastrointestinal tract and the normal method of defense is to create mucus.

Various bowel diseases occur after the bile has become too acid. Bile is created by the liver and flows to the gall bladder. All the bile that flows from the liver to the gall bladder has an alkaline pH. But after the bile leaves the gall bladder it can become very acid. Many people, in fact most people, are rapidly moving toward disease states and one of the steps toward disease occurs when they have lost the ability to maintain alkaline bile and acid bile develops. Under these conditions the body is forced to secrete abnormal amounts of the mucus to protect itself from acid.

Dr. Anderson claims at least ninety percent of the people who use his cleansing program have improved their health, increased their energy, and eliminated a large spectrum of disease conditions. This would seem to indicate that the elimination of mucoid plaque and the general cleansing that takes place removes a debilitating level of toxicity closely associated with loss of vitality and chronic disease.

Medical scientists have clearly stated they do not have all the answers. There is a great deal of guessing and concepts and facts are in a constant state of change. Most medical scientists avoid the word normal because "normal" implies that they know what is normal and what is not. Truth is, they really don't know.

With colon cancer it has been shown that the colonic epithelium (external layer) immediately adjacent to a colon cancer is thicker than normal. There is consideration that mucins affecting the mucosa are a field of pre-malignant tissue from which tumors arise. It is an agreed-upon medical concept that mucinogenic mucosa can be a transitional state that may develop into a more diseased condition in response to adjacent tumor or other pathologic condition.

Bile acids can stimulate mucosal and cell proliferation. The main reason bile becomes too acid is related to dietary ingestion of acid-forming foods - processed foods.

With Irritable Bowel Syndrome (IBS), mucus discharge upon defecation has been reported in approximately fifty percent of IBS patients. This supports the point that bowel irritation causes mucus to be secreted into the bowel as normal activity under stressful conditions. It is not uncommon for mucus to accumulate in any area of the body such as the gall bladder, arteries, urinary bladder, bronchials, etc.

Constipation is associated with bowel problems. It is also associated with poor diet; the same acid-forming diet that created the conditions that force the bowel to defend itself against acids and toxins by creating protective mucus. Constipation is common in the majority of IBS patients. Modern toilets aid in constipation.

Some gastroenterologists are aware of the concept of mucoid plaque. Abnormalities in colonic mucin glycoprotein are considered as potential subclinical markers for ulcerative colitis and possible other bowel diseases.

Bacteria and parasites are protected by mucoid plaque. Dr. Gibson and Dr. Macfarlane verified this point. They gave an example that E. Coli can be found completely separated from intestinal contents by a layer of mucin (mucoid plaque).

Dr. Bernard Jensen, DC, ND, Ph.D., made the following statement: "In the fifty years I've spent helping people to overcome illness, disability and disease, it has become crystal clear that poor bowel management lies at the root of most people's health problems." Dr. Jensen studied with many very successful doctors throughout the United States and Europe. He then built his own sanitarium and practiced with an open mind for over seventy years. His fame has traveled all over the world. He has even been nominated for the Nobel Prize.

In his book, *Tissue Cleansing Through Bowel Management*, Dr. Bernard Jensen describes mucoid plaque. "The heavy mucus coating in the colon thickens and becomes a host of putrefaction. The blood capillaries to the colon begin to pick up the toxins, poisons and noxious debris as it seeps through the bowel wall. All tissues and organs of the body are now taking on toxic substances. Here is the beginning of true autointoxication on a physiological level."

He goes on to say: "As we work with eliminating the encrusted mucus lining, we must also consider nourishing the new cells below it." And: "Bowel cleansing is an essential element in any lasting healing program. The toxic waste must be removed as quickly as possible to halt the downward spiral of failing health."

In the early 1900's, Dr. Tilden of Denver, Colorado, specialized in healing pneumonia, which was at that time the number one killer. During that time almost every doctor lost hundreds of their patients to that deadly plague. Dr. Tilden had more pneumonia cases than any other doctor and never lost a patient. He used no drugs at all. He simply cleaned out the colon (using enemas and colonics), used water therapy, and administered natural, live foods. Even in those days, his success was considered miraculous because other doctors were relying on drugs and continually meeting with failure.

Dr. Kellogg, MD of the Kellogg Sanitarium said: "Of the 22,000 operations that I have personally performed, I have never found a single normal colon, and of the 100,000 that were performed under my jurisdiction, not over six percent were normal." Dr. Kellogg said he knew of many cases in which operations were prevented by cleansing and revitalizing the bowel by eating alive food. He maintained that ninety percent of the diseases of civilization are due to improper function of the colon because of wrong eating habits and processed foods.

Dr. George C. Crile, head of the Crile Clinic in Cleveland and a well-known surgeon said: "There is no natural death. All deaths that come from so-called natural causes are merely the end point of progressive acid saturation. Many people go so far as to consider that sickness and disease are just a "cross" or an element that God gave them to bear here on earth. However, if they would take care of their body, and cleanse their colon and intestines, their problems would be pretty much eliminated and they could eliminate their "cross" by proper diet, proper exercise, and in general, proper living."

According to medical journals many doctors have proven over the years that the bowel is key to health or disease and the most important part of our physical anatomy to take care of in order to achieve successful healing.

Many believe today that all cancers, liver disorders, kidney, brain, and heart disorders receive their toxic malformations from the intestines. Sir Arbuthnot Lane, British Royal Surgeon, tried to make it clear when he wrote that he was "exceedingly impressed by the sequence of cancer and intestinal stasis." We know that changes in the breast caused by intestinal pollution have been described by many doctors.

Another author, Dr. Robert Gray, has described mucoid plaque in a manner similar to Dr. Jensen and Dr. Anderson. "Another type of constipation is present when old, hardened feces stick to the walls of the colon and do not pass out with the regular bowel movements." He continues: "Few people have any inkling as to how much old, hardened feces are chronically present with their bodies. As moisture is absorbed from a slimy medium in the colon the medium becomes sticky. As the medium is further dehydrated it becomes gluey and glues a coating of itself to the walls of the colon as it passes through. As layer after layer of gluey feces piles up in the colon they often form into a tough, rubbery black substance. Old feces may build up in pockets and they may coat the entire length of the colon and small intestines as well. They do not pass from the body with ordinary bowel movements but require special techniques to dissolve the glue that binds them in the body. Because non-mucoid material moves through the body quicker than mucoid material, the bowel tends to move two to three times per day when the intestines and colon are in non-mucoid condition."

He also discusses parasites. "They lodge themselves in the old matter that encrusts the walls of the intestinal tract. Without the presence of stagnant material to embed themselves in, intestinal parasites cannot maintain a foothold in the body. Remove this old, filthy, decaying mucoid matter and you will flush the parasites out as well." He explains mal-absorption in relation to mucoid plaque. "The accumulation of mucoid material along the walls of the small intestine can interfere with nutrient absorption even though nutritional intake may be adequate."

Dr. Jensen and Dr. Gray have different ideas as to how mucoid plaque is formed. Both of these authors felt that it was the mucus-forming foods and highly processed foods that contributed toward the formation of mucoid plaque. Dr. Anderson agrees they may contribute toward its composition, however his studies indicate that excess intake of acid-forming foods forces mucin to develop because it produces levels of acid the body cannot buffer due to electrolyte deficiency.

Dr. V.E. Irons, a pioneer in colon cleansing theory and activity, and a staunch advocate against modern medicine wrote a booklet titled: *The Destruction of Your Own Natural Protective Mechanism.* In this booklet he states: "The condition of the colons in this entire country are *far worse* than either the doctors, the AMA, the Drug houses, . . . or even the Natural Health industry have any conception . . . and believe in our theory that the *cause of most conditions of ill health is autointoxication* and that ninety-five percent of their troubles start in the colon." Could the cure be in the cause? Absolutely.

He goes on to give the reason why. "Because possibly ninety-nine percent of all ages and sexes have violated two of the major Natural Laws from one to three times every day since they were two years old. What are the two laws? 1. The *wrong* combination of foods. 2. The constant daily use of tremendous amounts of *dead foods.* The wrong application of both of these laws has caused the body's natural protective mechanism to secrete mucous into the colon to protect the body from absorbing the many poisons that those counterfeit foods create. But we have simply *overworked* Nature's protective mechanism to the point that the mechanism instead of protecting us from poisons now itself poisons us."

Unfortunately there has been little interest on this subject by the medical profession and theories vary from one end of the spectrum to the other. Medical science seems to be in denial to the experiences of tens of thousands of people. Medical science basically avoids admitting the mucoid theory and yet many thousands of people who first sought help from medical science ended up finding help from the natural procedures that modern medicine resists and denies. As modern medicine denied that Candidiasis was a cause to many illnesses for several decades after the alternative practitioners announced the problem, so does modern medicine deny the bowel problems in association with many diseases. They remain the "constipated profession" in the bowel as in the brain.

How unbelievably simple it is that the cure of colon problems and all others lies in the cause and all we have to do is to stop plugging it up with processed and lifeless foods.

This is just too simple to be true for most people that are complicated and don't want to be open-minded and dare to look to the cause. Many true doctors believe that by eliminating the debris from the bowel the mind will also become clearer in its thinking and if kept that way, enlightenment could occur.

Basic Parasite Information

Determining if there is parasite infection can be very difficult indeed. The subject has not received a great deal of attention and as such accurate testing methods are still being developed. However there are some facilities that specialize in parasitology. There will be an increased demand for effective testing procedures especially as awareness of the parasite problem begins to increase. Recent outbreaks resulting from the water supply of the upper mid-west will only expedite the development of parasitology. The outbreak mentioned was caused by Cryptosporidia, a microscopic parasite that infected thousands of people. Some died, especially those who had weakened immune systems. This is not the first time something like this has happened.

Symptoms associated with parasites include: anemia, hypoglycemia, indigestion, lack of energy, colitis, constipation, abdominal pain, back pain, headaches, acne and other skin problems, fever, blurred vision, pneumonia, cough, edema of face and eyes, poor assimilation, nausea, vomiting, ulcers, brain fog, weight loss and weakness, a feeling of fullness in the stomach, uncontrolled appetite, gas, and much more.

Some researchers state that the waste material produced by flukes (parasitic flatworms) is extremely carcinogenic and contributes to the formation of cancer. The waste material from just one tapeworm can make someone ill. Microscopic parasites can cause arthritis-like symptoms. Some call parasites "The Great Masqueraders."

I was telling a friend about tapeworms, how long they can get and how much they can drain and poison your body with their fecal debris. She asked if I had ever heard about the mail order weight-loss advertisements of the late 1920's. The pill was the head of a tapeworm that you would ingest and you would lose weight, among other things.

It is impossible to avoid all situations that could lead to parasitic infection. Here are two basic precautions that can serve as guidelines to follow:

1. *Eliminate criticism, judgment and complaining.* These nasty habits open the way for anger, resentment, fear and other negative emotions that ruin our immune systems and our health. Work on removing suppressed negative emotions.

2. *Cleanse the body and keep it clean on the inside.* Be a vegetarian and eat at least seventy-five percent raw foods.

Parasites are notoriously difficult to kill and/or expel from the body. Intestinal purification, through an ideal cleansing program, is the first and most important step to be taken. This powerful cleanse supports optimal internal health.

Many good doctors believe that everyone should do an ideal cleansing program at least once, and that everyone should also do some sort of parasite elimination program as well.

For more information on Dr. Anderson's cleansing programs, contact:

Arise & Shine
PO Box 1439
Mt. Shasta, CA 96067
(530) 926-0891
(800) 688-2444
FAX (530) 926-8866

John Cotton has successfully helped over seven thousand people get healthy through cleansing with Dr. Anderson's formulas. For body cleanses, please contact him at: (510) 653-5050 or www.thefirewithin.com.

Hydrated Bentonite

One of the first items to include in an herbal "first aid kit" would be hydrated Bentonite. Bentonite is known for its highly absorptive properties and its ability to draw out and bind heavy metals, drugs and other toxins form the body. This clay has been used for thousands of years as both an internal and external purification aid. The Egyptians used it to preserve their famous mummies. The ancient Greeks and Romans used it to restore health. The great German Naturopaths of the last century hailed clay as one of Nature's great remedies. Mahatma Ghandi advocated the use of clay for health and purification. Numerous so-called "primitive" tribes have used clay for both internal and external purification.

Today Bentonite clay is increasingly used both internally and externally by those interested in natural remedies and it is included on the FDA's famous "GRASS" list, which stands for "Generally Recognized As Safe". With increasing public knowledge about minerals some have expressed concern over the presence of small amounts of aluminum in Bentonite clay. However there have been numerous hair analyses done on those who use the clay that indicate the body does not absorb aluminum from Bentonite.

Bentonite is one of the volcanic ashes. It is not a drug or chemical composition made in a laboratory. It is a product of Mother Earth. Bentonite in ages past was blown into the sky by volcanic actions which sifted down to help impregnate the soil with its twenty-five to thirty-five trace minerals. Bentonite, under a high-power microscope is seen as extremely minute rectangular particles, similar in shape to a business card. When hydrated it generates and maintains a very strong electromagnetic field which allows it to attract and hold unwanted, non-nutritive substances such as pesticides and other toxins so that they can be eliminated from the body.

Dr. Jensen suggests using Bentonite to absorb radiation from the bones. Since so many of us are subject to various forms of radiation, whether from x-rays or televisions or computers, this would be something to consider. This could be extremely important for those who have undergone radiation treatment for cancer. Some people take about a cup of extra thick liquid Bentonite and put it into their bath water. It is highly effective in drawing out toxins. But too much or too long an exposure will dry out the skin.

Some Bentonite users report relief from swelling, pain and aching in the gums and teeth. Since these symptoms are manifestations of toxins or infections in the tissue surrounding the teeth and gums, it is easily apparent that Bentonite's powerful absorbing qualities would provide relief for these areas. Those suffering from pain or swelling in the teeth and gum area are advised to take a psyllium shake several times a day to absorb any poisons being released from the infected area into the bowel. In this situation it would also help to pack powdered Bentonite directly onto the swollen, painful areas to draw the irritating toxins out. A combination of powdered Bentonite and plantain (another powerful absorber) can be used in a square of cheesecloth or muslin which is then dampened and placed over the irritated area of the gums. This seems to work best if you do this before bed and sleep with it under your lips.

Hydrated Bentonite is invaluable for skin eruptions as well. Dr. Anderson once got an extremely severe case of poison oak in every nook and cranny of his body after a camping trip. When he got home he put thick hydrated Bentonite on every spot he saw or felt and noticed immediate relief from the itchiness. However, the next morning after showering it off, he saw that there were still some red spots and the itchiness returned. Again he applied hydrated Bentonite and again the itchiness left. This time when he showered it all off, it was completely gone!

Many have used a paste of hydrated Bentonite as a facial mask for general skin enlivening and cleansing, as well as for specific skin eruptions. Whenever applied to a pimple or infected skin bump the hydrated Bentonite will simply draw out the toxic matter that is causing the eruption. This application should be repeated each night before retiring until the skin eruption has been completely eliminated.

In the *Medical Annals of the District of Columbia*, Vol. 20, No. 6, June 1961, under the title "The Value of Bentonite for Diarrhea," are the results of the clinical work performed by a team of medical doctors using hydrated Bentonite in the treatment of diarrhea. The diarrhea was the result of virus infections, food allergies, spastic colitis and food poisoning. The results of the scientific investigation indicated that liquid Bentonite provided substantial relief in ninety-four percent of the cases. The percent of relief indicated by the symptoms were: abdominal cramps eighty percent, anorexia seventy-eight percent, malaise eighty percent, headaches seventy-one percent, nausea eighty-five percent, and weakness one hundred percent. The article concluded: "By virtue of its physical action, Bentonite serves as an absorbent aid in detoxification of the intestinal canal."

Both the *US Government Bureau of Mines Booklet* #609 and a late edition of the *Dispensary of the United States of America*, an official compendium, give Bentonite high praise: "In addition to the growing number of external uses for Bentonite, it has been reported to be of value as an intestinal evacuant when used in the form of a gel."

Since Bentonite has such strong absorptive powers some may be concerned about whether it might absorb necessary nutrients from the alimentary canal as well. Independent experiments designed to find out how much this absorption would adversely affect the growth and health of animals indicated no ill effects when the intake of Bentonite was twenty-five percent of the total diet, but did adversely affect the health of the animals when the intake of Bentonite was increased to fifty percent of the total diet. But even twenty-five percent of the total diet is a *lot* of Bentonite!

It is important however, not to take any nutritional supplement at the same time as the Bentonite. Especially when used with psyllium the Bentonite will absorb anything of nutritional value such as herbs, friendly bacteria, vitamins, as wells as toxins, bad bacteria and parasites. Be sure to wait one and a half to two hours after doing a Bentonite shake before taking anything nutritional.

Scientific research has shown that Bentonite's absorptive

action is due to five characteristics. First, it has a large and varied mineral content. Second, it has a negative electrical attraction for positive-charged particles. Third, its particles (being shaped like calling cards) have the wide surfaces negative-polarized and the edges positive-polarized, which give it an incredible negative pulling power. Forth, the very minuteness of the particles of Bentonite gives a large surface area in proportion to the volume used, thus enabling it to pick up many times its own weight in positively charged particles. Fifth, to obtain maximum effectiveness in the human body, it must be put in a liquid colloidal-gel state.

Though Bentonite has been used internally by Native Americans for hundreds of years to help detoxify the bowels, modern practitioners recommend that when using it internally always use it with psyllium, as a psyllium shake. The reason for this is that Bentonite contains inorganic minerals and psyllium helps to prevent undesirable inorganic minerals from entering the system.

Other uses of Bentonite which are documented by Jason R. Eaton, a researcher of the living clay include:

EXTERNAL:

Bone and muscle damage due to accidents, sports injuries, etc.
Carpal Tunnel Syndrome, Tendonitis
Healing of internal organs
High blood pressure
Chronic headaches
Skin conditions (acne, eczema, rashes and more)
Rapid healing of injuries (bruises, sprains, burns, etc.)
Severe bacterial infections (gangrene, etc.)
Muscular imbalance (tension, chronic pain, stress)
Skin rejuvenation and deep cleansing
Radiation

INTERNAL:

Detoxification of body/digestive system (bacterial, organic and non-organic toxins)
Elimination of internal parasites
Immune system (fixes free oxygen in the blood steam, increases T-cell count, fights free radicals)
Mercury poisoning
Trace mineral supplement
Liver detoxification (improves many joint troubles and conditions)
Stomach aches

These uses are further documented by author Michael Abehsera in his book, *Amazing Cures from the Earth Itself: The Healing Clay*.

What's so nice about Nature-made material is that it has been around forever and people have been using it, and it works. Where man-made drugs (chemicals) can have a deadly effect and it may cause some sort of damage or side-effect, besides it accumulates and gets stored in the tissue because the body does not recognize it and it could be passed on to new generations. Like lead, mercury, aluminum and many other chemicals and elements that we use today in vaccinations, drugs, pesticides, etc. Nature does the healing if we eliminate an unnatural lifestyle.

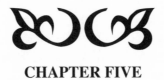

CHAPTER FIVE

What's <u>really</u> wrong today and how can we fix it naturally?

"The history of mankind is an immense sea of errors in which a few obscure truths may here and there be found."
Cesare Beccaria

We are now on dangerous ground. There is visible damage to the human race and more yet invisible. We are getting weaker and more vulnerable than ever before. In just the last one hundred years we've brought about a situation nearing total disaster. The warning signs are everywhere, yet we ignore them. We are too preoccupied to see and by being unaware, bring about our own destruction. The future of the next few generations is very uncertain even for the ones in the best of circumstances.

"When a man's science exceeds his sense, he perishes by his own ignorance."

Asian proverb

The human race has endured and flourished through mental strength because their physical was more in harmony with Nature. Only the fittest survive, yet it is wrong to measure only mental capacity in considering a person's degree of success in financial or academic circles. More important and a more reliable indicator is the state of their physical health and their outlook on and philosophy of life. What good is money when you cannot buy health at any price? Why die of cancer or some other illness that could have been avoided or prevented? The fittest will survive.

Intelligent is what we become only when our innate wisdom seeks the truth. Today we are poorly informed and sadly ignorant. The increased health problems are but a reflection of that ignorance.

Our leaders, schools, food industries, medical professionals, and pharmaceutical companies, every bit as uniformed, need to wake up! Time is running out. Senseless delay can cost you your health - life and unwillingness to change will cause incredible disasters . . . and ultimately our destruction. We have been on this planet the shortest time and yet have done the most damage. For an optimist, I am concerned.

"If I could live my life over again, I would devote it to proving that germs seek their natural habitat, diseased tissue, rather than being the cause of diseased tissue."
Dr. Rudolph Virchow

The confused medical obsession with germs, viruses, antibiotics, prescription drugs, and treating symptoms is nothing but clear ignorance. Misguided, drug-oriented institutions are extremely dangerous to humans, animals, and the health and well being of our shared planet.

We must free the medical profession from its dogma and unawareness. It could happen. Many are slowly adopting the idea of natural, healthy nutrition and lifestyle.

In the meantime, millions have died unnecessarily and millions more will die because of faulty beliefs and the unwillingness to face reality. There is a place for modern medicine and new technology but not in treating disease. We didn't depend on them for thousands of years. What damage has been done in the last one hundred?

"In nature there are neither rewards or punishments, there are consequences."
Robert Ingersoll

We must obey the fundamental laws of Nature. Obsessed with superiority of science and technology, we disregard the simple wisdom Nature offers as beneath notice. Obedience to Nature's wisdom equals life itself. Health, happiness, harmony, love, success, and liberty. All in one!

People are too clever for their own good. They will do anything and everything to pursue progress and pleasure - at any cost. At the same time they sow the seeds of their own destruction and that of innocent others, without ever noticing or being aware of what they've done. That's not intelligence. That is not awareness.

"Unless the doctors of today become the dietitians of tomorrow, the dietitians of today will become the doctors of tomorrow."
                                                    Dr. Alexis Carrel, in 1936

Since we are what we eat, and what we can absorb, nutrition is the most important factor in our health and survival. Foods of today are processed and manufactured, extremely depleted of nutritional value. In that state they hamper the body and cannot heal it. Poor nutrition = empty calories = starvation.

Today's foods are grounds for various deficiencies that cause disease and destruction of normal body processes. Disease in fact is caused by a biochemical insufficiency of the body, and the way we prepare food. We kill the food with heat before we eat it. Much of today's food is genetically engineered.

Our bodies become breeding grounds for bacteria, our blood becomes toxic and sticky, therefore it cannot properly supply the organs with what it needs and degeneration occurs under a different name for each organ affected.

For example protein is acid-forming in the body. The body in order to keep normal pH balance has to borrow calcium from bones to neutralize the acid. The more protein we eat the more calcium must be released from the bones into the bloodstream in order to keep the body's balance alkaline. The eventual outcome is osteoporosis, among many other degenerative conditions.

How does modern medicine treat osteoporosis? With drugs and an extra calcium pill added to the diet, hormone (estrogen) therapy and surgical repair of broken bones.

What is the natural solution? Eat *less* protein and keep the blood naturally more alkaline with proper nutrition through eating more green, leafy vegetables, raw and organic.

We have no choice but to go back to Nature in order to correct health problems. Proper nutrition, lots of organic raw fruits and vegetables in their original form, is a cure for any ailment - **true** medicine!

In looking over the whole process consider that disease is an eliminative activity of the body. The body is constantly trying to remain well and disease can be looked upon as a "cure". By allowing the disease to run its course we're giving the body every opportunity to recover of its own accord.

Fever is good. It is there to save your life. What suffering mankind must go through before the truth can be recognized. Why, when the truth is so obvious?

"Our body is a machine for living. It is organized for that, it is its nature. Let life go on in it unhindered and let it defend itself, it will do more than if you paralyze it by encumbering it with remedies."

Leo Tolstoy, *War and Peace*

We have found ways to overcome symptomatic disease, yet we are developing more chronic diseases than ever before. Twenty-five years ago only one out of every twenty-five people had cancer. Today the number is one in three. Disease is handled from the inside out. Cleansing always proceeds from the inside out.

Disease is the consequence of bad habits and wrong living. When diseases become apparent they should be given a chance to eliminate themselves.

If you become constipated don't use laxatives. If you have a burning stomach don't use an antacid. If pollen is causing you trouble don't take shots. These are quick-fix patches. This is how chronic and degenerative diseases develop over time. Trying to fix the symptoms with medication won't work. It drives it in deeper.

All diseases are curable but not every patient is!

What prevents a disease will also cure it. The cure is found in prevention-cause.

Theory amounts to very little if we cannot find a way to back it up with practical means. They must work hand in hand or the theory must change.

We know now that our diet is the main contributor to our well being or degenerative conditions. So we must become more aware of what we put in our body. The purer and simpler we keep it the easier it is on our body and the longer our life span will be. Think about it. In order to correct the problem we need to know what the cause is. Can you hear that? Could it possibly be any simpler than that?

Simple diet is the key and best for the body in order to keep it clean and debris free.

"Nothing will benefit human health or increase the chance for survival of life on earth as will the evolution to a vegetarian diet."

Albert Einstein

Can you imagine if that vegetarian diet is all raw/organic? We would realize that we all have Albert Einstein in us. We would use more than ten percent of our brain. Heaven on earth in all aspects of our lives. Love, enlightenment, an incredible awareness. I truly believe that we would not get involved in other people's business and wars would not make sense to us. We would see no need to depend on any bureaucratic agency for anything, the truth would be obvious, there would be nothing to hide. We would be honest and more respectful of our fellow man and our planet earth.

There are many differences in human behavior and diet plays the biggest role. I studied people on natural diets and can honestly say that they are calmer, kinder, more loving and most importantly clear thinking. Without prejudice, the confusion we are in today is mainly due to our nutrition. Everything else is secondary.

In order to fix what's wrong we have to be aware that there is something wrong and investigate, then remove that which is wrong. There is no other way.

The reason why doctors are so arrogant today and pretend to be gods is due to antibiotics and quick fixes. Now antibiotics do not work any longer because of the damage (consequences) they've done to our immune system. Ultimately they are being forced to look to the true cause yet they are so attached to their old ways.

Sun, air and water

"The course of nature is the art of God."
Edward Young

"Nothing has such a power to broaden the mind as the ability to investigate systematically and truly all that comes under observation in life."
Marcus Aurelius Antonius

There are three principles of cure:

1) A healthy blood stream for healthy cell structure (raw/organic nutrition)
2) The blood circulating rapidly enough to supply cell structure with all necessary building elements to build and repair as required. With natural minerals and elements and proper elimination of the dead cells to keep the blood clean.
3) Rest. Gravity is least detrimental when the body is lying in a prone position. Rest allows the body to recuperate and regenerate. Tiredness is a barometer and fatigue, the first symptom of disease.

Iridology immediately reveals in which part of the body concentrated trouble exists and the condition of the organ affected. Cure is dependent upon the cleansing of body tissue and replacing old tissue with new. All cure starts from within out, from the head down and in the reverse order the symptoms appeared. This is Hering's Law of Cure and how it works. The last thing (illness) that surfaces will be the first thing that gets cured and the first thing (illness) that surfaces will be the last to be cured. This all takes time and when it surfaces it is called a healing crisis.

Don't expect a quick fix. It took time to get where we are, so it will take time to reverse it. Be patient. Be in touch with the earth, sun, and fresh air.

Humans are shallow breathers at rest but that isn't always sufficient to get enough oxygen into our lungs and from there to our bloodstream. It also isn't always enough to rid our lungs of all the toxic residue of breathing, carbon dioxide. If you don't do some form of exercise on a regular basis, at least remember to walk and take deep cleansing breaths several times a day. Read Dr. Bragg's book listed in the index on proper breathing.

Be in touch with Nature. Quench your thirst with fresh fruits that have organic water in them. The minerals in tap water are collected from the ground and are inorganic. They cannot be assimilated by the body unless they are chelated or bound with organic molecules as they are in fresh fruits and vegetables. Eat plenty of the fresh stuff and if you need water, drink distilled with no inorganic minerals, toxic chemicals, and other elements. When distilled water enters the body, it will pick up mineral deposits accumulated in the joints, artery walls, kidneys, or wherever such deposits occur, and begin to carry them back out. Little by little you will notice you are more flexible and moveable. Your arteries will gradually become more elastic and your blood pressure more normal. Distilled water attracts inorganic material, while organic materials stays in the tissues where they need to be. Hard water carries inert materials into the body and distilled water carries them out. Simple.

We must remove all the sludge. The body will become supple and ageless, the joints, arteries, cells and nerve tracts will be free of inorganic mineral deposits.

In the old days, we used to drink rainwater (natural, distilled water). Every house had a cistern. Today we have acid rain and pollution. Think about it. Other than raw fruits and fresh juices, distilled water is the best for you. Put a twist of lemon or orange in the water to balance the pH.

For more information on water call or write: THE CHOICE IS CLEAR, Acres USA, 10227 E. 61st St., Raytown, MS 64133, 816-737-0064.

Hydrotherapy, hot baths, and hot springs have been used for centuries to heal people. They cleanse the biggest organ (skin) and pull debris out of the pores. Enjoy hot springs and baths whenever you can. Check the internet for locations of hot springs and mud baths. They are very therapeutic, relaxing and excellent for your health.

"We choose the god-like splendor of the best-loved Sun to inspire us; may the shining Sun brighten your life!"
Ramayana

All life on this planet derives from the sun. The sun beats like a great heart through every living organism. Science even says the molecules that make up our bodies were born in the great inferno of our sun.

The air we breathe is transformed energy from the sun. Plants absorb the energy and transform carbon dioxide (CO2) into the oxygen (O2) all animals need to breathe. Animal respiration depends specifically on solar energy.

The foods we eat are energy reservoirs of transformed solar energy. Through photosynthesis, plants capture energy from the sun and lock that power into their stems, leaves, seeds, roots, and fruits. All animals are transformed plants. The body of a gazelle is nothing more than grass. The body of a cheetah is, therefore, by extension through its prey, also grass.

We are beings nourished directly by sun's energy. Sunlight can transform your health. The human body with many capillaries in the skin surface, draws in sunlight, and hemoglobin converts it directly into nourishment, just as chlorophyll does in plants. Hemoglobin contains iron and chlorophyll contains magnesium. Otherwise they're identical.

The sun makes us cheerful and light-hearted. It cultivates a healthy, positive attitude. Lack of sunlight has the opposite effect. People in more northern climates are often afflicted by a seasonal depression (SADD) attributed to lack of sunshine in winter months. Today people spend most of their time indoors.

The benefits of sunshine are improved by eating the correct diet. Sun and fresh air act like magnets to draw toxins to the skin surface. The skin is the body's largest eliminative organ and proper exposure to the sun is a great way to get rid of that waste.

Since elements like Beta-carotene in green leafy vegetables can help protect your skin from ultraviolet radiation, good nutrition allows you longer exposure to sunlight without raising the risk of skin cancer. In fact a diet high in animal fat, chemicals, and low in green leafy vegetables has been positively linked to skin cancer. Free radicals and toxins in unprotected skin are cooked and mutated by ultraviolet rays.

"Cholesterol [the good kind] *turns to vitamin D - a vitamin needed for proper bone formation - when sunlight or ultraviolet light strikes the skin. Without this vitamin the bones do not become calcified and will bend easily. This condition is called rickets."*

Dr. Kime, *Sunlight*

Sunlight builds the immune system and increases skin's oxygenation. Sunlight also lowers blood sugar. A diet high in natural fruit sugar must also include sunshine on the skin to help metabolize that sugar. Sunshine helps store sugar as glycogen in the liver, muscles and cells for later use.

The sun stimulates capillaries under the skin and brings more blood to the surface to help heal bruises, cuts, and rashes. Fungus is destroyed by direct sunlight. Sunshine aids digestion, improves eyesight, and regulates hormones. Our eyes need sunlight every day to reset our internal clocks but never, ever look directly into the sun or you might do irreparable damage to your retinas.

Commercial sunscreens impair the body's natural sunburn alarm. Most lotions, creams, and butters are made of chemicals and animal fats that produce cancer-causing free radicals. The best protection from ultraviolet radiation comes from the inside. Eat lots of organic raw, green leafy vegetables and fresh fruit and try fresh aloe vera juice as a substitute sun lotion. Even so, watch your exposure.

Beware though. Artificial light is not the same as sunlight. Many endocrine fluids suffer when we are exposed to artificial light, especially at night. Light at the wrong time of day confuses the body; pituitary and pineal glands trigger the thyroid to pull more calcium from the bones causing thyroid problems and also near-sightedness. People who leave lights on at night may develop other problems. This is not natural.

Taking the melatonin hormone is potentially dangerous. One way you can increase your melatonin hormone is to make certain you sleep in an absolutely dark room. Do not turn on any lights as they will suppress your own body's melatonin production. Melatonin is natural hormone that is only made in complete darkness. So if you are depressed or cannot sleep, pay attention to how much exposure to artificial light you get so you don't confuse your body. Why go against Nature?

Let Nature take its course. Before the sun goes down try to finish work that requires light. Do not leave night-lights on for children. Try to teach them to go to sleep when it gets dark. The rest that we get before midnight is more important that the rest you receive after even if you sleep in late in the morning. Do it right from the start and you won't have sick children. Their intuition will work better if they are in tune with Nature.

Sensory Awareness

"These workshops are not discussion, but practice. The approach is through the organism as a whole - the living totality in which all our faculties arise. The actual experience of exploring, freeing, and deepening our innate potential can, if we follow it through, have far-reaching consequences in all spheres of living."

Charlotte Selver

"In order to live and die without regret, we must be true to what each moment asks of us. This means going beyond the tasks that all too often consume our days; and living with a more acute awareness. Sensory Awareness is a mindfulness practice that invites us to trust our own innate responsiveness. Through paying attention to our sense, to breathing, to the natural forces that are always with us . . . we can begin to let go of hindrances and habits that constrict us, becoming more truly available for what our lives offer and ask of us."

Lee Klinger Lesser

I must mention my one hundred year old mentor and friend, Charlotte Selver. She holds workshops around the world on the subject of awareness and purpose. The late psychologist and author Erich Fromm says of her workshops: "I know Charlotte Selver's work, having studied with her for several years. I have found it of greatest help for myself. I consider the principles on which this work is based of great significance for the full unfolding of the personality."

The late Alan W. Watts, author and philosopher said: "Charlotte conveys the actual sensation of some of the things which I try to express in mere words - and above all, the organic relationship of man with the whole world of Nature."

"The work of Charlotte Selver . . . is the inner experience of entire being, the pure flow of sensory awareness when the mind through calmness ceases to work - deeper than mind-made awareness. What is this "entire being?" If you want to say something about it, you should know how to be it." - Shunryu Suzuki Roshi

The Esalen Institute wrote: "Ms. Selver's more than 50 years of pioneering work in the United States has been the basis for most of the work with sensory awareness, sensory awakening and related approaches which are now gaining wide acceptance."

For more on Charlotte Selver and her work, contact the Sensory Awareness Foundation, 955 Vernal Avenue, Mill Valley, CA 94941. I also recommend reading the book *Sensory Awareness: The Rediscovery of Experiencing*, by Charles V. W. Brooks, Charlotte's beloved husband.

At one hundred years young, Charlotte Selver still practices, teaching her work to new students all across the US, Mexico, and Europe.

Don't miss the opportunity to meet this enlightened human being and experience her gifts. It might just be that her presence will click something within you and you'll never be the same. It happened to me.

"We experience expansion as awareness, understanding or whatever. When we are completely aware we have a feeling of being one with all life. Then, and only then we have no resistance to other beings. It is timeless bliss, with no limits, only perceptions and feelings. Love in action that is available to every being in the universe all the time."

Thaddeus Golas

Vibratory theory or trigger response

"Let no one presume to give advice to others that has not first given good advice to himself."

Seneca

Diet has a definite vibratory effect on the body. We become aware of disease through the nervous system which is highly attuned to whatever is going on in the body. Due to the intimate communication between the brain and every cell of the body, vibratory response in harmony in either body or mind is bound to be mutually interactive.

Coffee addiction is bad for you. The beneficial effects of various treatments are neutralized almost immediately after the intake of caffeine. Drug vibrations affect the mind and most of all the body.

The body is built of everything the universe is built of. We can go far in our imagination when we consider the similarities in the nature of light radiation and nerve impulses. Light radiation and nerve impulses are made of the same stuff. Disease comes into existence through abnormal vibrations. Every disease has its own symptoms, its own calling, its own craving, its own appetite, and yet they are one with all. These conditions are expressed in the form of vibratory rates. Live food has a higher vibration.

In working with vibratory action we increase the vital energy of the body by using health-building methods. The activity for health will overcome the activity of disease. If the factors that are breaking down the vital health of the body are being fed (coffee, drugs, sugar), you can readily see without any trouble how chronic disease can be developed. To break down chronic disease, starve the disease. It must not be given a chance to exist. Build vital energy and healthy respiratory activities into the body and eventually health will be the result.

Native Americans believe the Earth does not belong to man. *"Man belongs to the Earth. All things are connected, like blood ties which unite a family. Man does not weave the web of life; he is only a strand in it. Whatever happens to the Earth, happens to all of us. Whatever man does to the web of life, he does to himself."*

Neither drugs nor vitamins are a cure for anything. The body heals itself. The human body is incredibly intelligent. It usually responds to intelligent therapies and the healing professional can help this process by offering intelligent therapies.

Dr. Schulze puts it nicely: *"True healing comes from creating a lifestyle that is healthy. Stopping the things you did that made you sick, and beginning a new program of health and wellness. Your body will completely heal itself. It has the intelligence, it just needs your cooperation.*

"All disease is caused by some type of blockage, whether it is circulatory, lymphatic, digestive, nutritional, eliminative, emotional, or whatever. When you free the blockage and let the energy flow, healing comes in.

"Tomorrow's health is built on what you do today!

"We need to know that our healing and our freedom can only come from true knowledge and our willingness to trust, to believe again, and to love. Somehow we've lost our way."

Use your intuition as guidance and listen to what you hear. Nature is harmony and man is a part of Nature. Man himself must be harmonic. The laws governing mind and body reflect and partake of the functioning of greater Nature.

For each of us, there comes a time to let go. You will know when that time has come. When you have done all you can do it is time to detach. Deal with your feelings. Face your fears about losing control. Gain control of yourself and your own responsibilities. Free others to be who they are. In doing so you will set yourself free.

We are always so careful to see that no one gets hurt. No one, that is, but ourselves. "Your wish is my command. Your problem is my problem." We are caretakers. Rescuing is enabling - a destructive form of healing. We rescue any time we take responsibility for another human being and enable that person to not have to fend for himself. Doing things for that person, speaking for him, solving any problems. Doing something for someone, though that person is perfectly capable of doing it himself.

Live and let live. Use your intuition as a guide and listen to what you hear. Good thoughts and good food are good medicine.

We know that no one can cure anybody or anything without knowing the cause. So to understand any disease it is necessary to know the cause. We know that toxemia is the cause of all disease. What then causes toxemia is curing the body of enervated damage. In order to get well, we must then know how to stay well and what caused our ill health. How can, then, any doctor cure any disease without pointing out to the patient his bad habits and enervated body and mind. No one can cure anything without removing the cause.

"Nothing ever just happens. Everything happens just."
Dr. Bernard Jensen

Raw diet has a vibratory effect on our body. We become harmonized when we eat food that is alive. Enzymes in food that are alive help digest nutrients better. When we eat cooked food enzymes are killed by heat so our body has to manufacture more of its own digestive enzymes to utilize and process that food. The vibrational energy disappears with heat and cooking puts strain on the organs and digestion allowing the disease to set in. When the body no longer manufactures enzymes to carry out all bodily functions and needs, life ceases.

The *Mandala* as point of departure

"It is only under ideal conditions, when life is still simple and unconscious enough to follow the serpentine path of instinct without hesitation or misgiving, that the compensating function of the unconscious works with entire success. The more civilized and complicated a man is, the less he is able to follow his instincts. His complicated living conditions and the influence of his environment are so strong that they drown the quiet voice of nature. Opinions, beliefs, theories and collective tendencies appear in its stead and back up all the aberrations of the conscious mind . . . "

Carl Jung

I totally agree with Carl Jung, Nature is simple and her laws of cause and effect are immutable. When we stay in touch with Nature we can more easily follow our instincts. That quiet little voice of Nature is always a true answer for us. So to know the right answer, we have to ask the right question. In order to do that, we have to be in tune with the divine.

So is it really luck? I think not. Like I mentioned many times before, even miracles have a cause (reason behind them). Harmony and balance are always present even when you think that you are not.

The nice thing about it is that you, too, can reach that point of harmony and balance just by knowing and being aware of it. My English has no words to express the way I feel it inside. Some that know what I mean may perhaps understand. You that do are needed to get this message across.

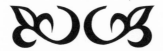

CHAPTER SIX
How to change the way you eat

"Change is not made without inconvenience, even from worse to better."

Richard Hooker

When your life force is exhausted, then there is death. No matter what kind of health problem you have, you have to realize that the doctor, surgery, drugs, chemotherapy or radiation or any other technique will not heal your body. If you do not look to the cause and if you do not give the body vital force (live nutrients) then the body will not heal itself. But when you do, only then the body will heal.

I have seen people banish ill health by eating nothing but raw fruits for breakfast. For the noon meal, a raw vegetable salad, chopped or grated cabbage, carrots or beets, etc). You can add any other raw vegetables you desire (lettuce, cucumber, radishes, avocados, tomatoes, herbs, sprouts, etc). Start slowly so that the intestines can clean out all the debris and mucous. If this diet does not agree with you, it means that you have a sick bowel. You will notice that it will agree with you as you clean out the walls of the sick bowel. It took a long time for the bowel to get to this stage and it will take a while to get better and it will. These raw salads are Mother Nature's cleanser-broom. As you get better with this salad you can have some lightly steamed vegetables or baked squash or sweet potato). Don't worry about concentrated protein. It's a myth and you're hooked on it. You can have some fish if you must, but if you want to cure your serious problems, I would advise organic vegetable protein (nuts and seeds, wheat germ, tofu, brown rice, beans, etc). They do not have uric acid to clog your arteries. Meat is a second hand food. An animal ate the green, growing plant that produced the meat and you saw earlier how hard it is to break it down. It is a fact that vegetarians live healthier, longer lives. Allow yourself at least four or five hours between each meal and eat only when hungry. When I ask ill people if they like raw salads, they usually say they do not because it gives them gas. Many like salad dressing and eat salads only because of the dressings. The dressing might be the culprit of their ill health.

Eat organic fresh fruits and vegetables as often as possible. Raw is imperative. You must realize that this is not a fad, cult or some new religion. This is a fact that will improve, extend and achieve your optimum health and life span. The enzymes in raw food play a role of life versus death. Enzymes accomplish all biological work and functions that are in the cells of every living body, plant and animal. In other words, we would not be alive if it wasn't for enzymes. So raw food is a must because cooked (dead) food is enzyme-less and creates an acidic state and disease.

When you feel hungry use a variety of fresh raw sauces that can be used for dips or dressings. Salads can be your main dish. By using a variety of dressings, you won't grow tired of the same flavor. You can create a salad to suit each member of the family as easily as making one large salad. Place little piles of vegetables, fruit, sprouts, and seeds in each individual dish then pour on the dressing or dip of choice. Shred, chop, slice, blend, or mix tomatoes, radishes, avocados, celery, carrots, cucumbers, grapes, onions, or whatever, the way each person likes it as a base for the salad. The juices and the dressing run down into the main ingredients and are especially tasty when you get to them. You can also use fruit like sliced oranges, apples, peaches, and seeds or nuts to add flavor, texture and color.

Any vegetables you don't like to eat, you will like if you juice them.

Sprouts are great. You should include them in your salads. Alfalfa, chickpea or garbanzo, mung bean, lentil, aduki, and fenugreek sprouts are all great combined together or on their own. And don't forget to sprinkle chives, garlic, dill, pepper, herbs, spices, seeds or nuts on top. Be creative. Have fun! I make things up as I go and based on whatever ingredients I have available at the time. The tools you'll need are a food processor, Vita Mix (blender) and a juicer, a garlic press, shredder and coffee grinder.

When you experiment with different techniques for

chopping, grating or slicing a variety of vegetables and fruits you will never run out of ideas. When the veggies are finely sliced, they're juicier and more flavorful. Take a look at some of my favorite dressings that will make any salad "finger-licking" good.

Salads are meals unto themselves. They are great for dieters and anyone who likes to graze or snack between meals. You will be pleasantly surprised how filling and satisfying salads truly are.

When I took Dr. Schulze's class he fed us for a week on "rainbow salad" with garlic olive oil and ginger dressing mixed with a touch of Bragg's apple cider vinegar. The plates were huge. That's all we ate for a week and never craved anything else. On the last day, Dr. Schulze told us we were going to have a surprise for dinner. Mealtime came and we were served the same salad with the same dressing but on the side was a huge, organic baked potato. Something so simple, yet we were all delighted!

The more used to raw you get, the bigger the variety you can have. As it gets colder you can have baked squash or pumpkin with your salad. Better yet, shred a raw one with a fine shredder or food processor and add to the salad.

My favorite raw sweet potato salad is so satisfying you can only eat a small portion, but you'll feel good all day.

When you eat food that is raw and natural, you do not crave very much, rather only what your body needs. You cannot possibly overeat. It would be very difficult to eat too much fruit, salad or a particular vegetable. When you eat processed food it is easy to overeat and get stuffed because the body does not get satisfied when the enzymes are lacking, so you always crave more hoping that you will ingest proper and needed enzymes.

Recipes:

Raw Sweet Potato Salad

Shred an organic sweet potato, skin and all, with a shredder. Quickly add some orange or lemon juice so the potato doesn't darken. Add finely chopped celery and onions, parsley, raisins, walnuts, apples (and anything else you might like). Dress with fresh orange juice, olive or flax seed oil, a pinch of Celtic sea salt or *Bragg Liquid Aminos* (available in health food stores), and mix well. Enjoy, chewing each bite slowly. You can use any dressing of your choice, too. Be creative. You can't mess up!

Tahini Dressing or Dip

Grind a cup of sesame seeds in a blender or food processor. Add the fresh juice of an orange or lemon (if you want it thicker for a dip, use less juice; thinner, use more juice). Add herbs for a green salad, or fruit for a fruit salad. The sky's the limit. If you want variety, try honey, dates, raisins, prunes, figs, lemon, garlic, chives, cayenne pepper, basil, parsley, rosemary, or any flavors you like. Use your imagination. If you don't like the result, change ingredients until you find a combination that suits you!

Nut or Seed Dressings and Dips

Nuts and seeds are especially great in the wintertime when your body needs extra calories to keep you warm. Remember, they are all acidic. You can prepare the nuts (almonds, walnuts, sunflower seeds, pine nuts, etc.) first by soaking them in water overnight so they are more easily digested and absorbed, then grind them up.

If you're making a dip, add less juice or water to your recipe. For a dressing, use more to make it pour easier. The secret with nuts is to make certain they're fresh and grinding them smooth. If you're making a desert, add fresh vanilla, coconut, and any fresh fruit in season. A dip for vegetables, add spices and different seasonings with a touch of your favorite herbs. Make up your own name for each dip or dressing! Have fun.

Banana Delight

Finely grind sesame seeds in a blender. Mix them with fresh orange juice and a little lemon. Add in a few ripe bananas. It helps if the bananas are cold before blending them. Put in a glass bowl. Take a mango and blend it separately. Pour over the sesame/banana mix. You can use a variety of other fruits like ripe strawberries, cantaloupe, cherries, or berries. Try different combinations! This can be your main dish if you juice some fresh vegetables an hour before you eat your banana delight.

Banana Sundae

Cut a cool ripe banana in half lengthwise and lay on a plate. Sprinkle with freshly ground walnuts. Place fresh strawberries on top (or any other fresh fruit in season), and squeeze some fresh orange juice over the fruit. For more flavor, try adding a touch of maple syrup or honey.

Tomato Dressing

Chop a few tomatoes into a blender. Add some garlic, basil, olive oil, and blend. Mix in some capers or dill, and pour over your favorite salad. You can make this dressing with any vegetable you love, just add different herbs to change the flavor. This is best when tomatoes are in season.

Shakes to Live For

Soak almonds overnight in water, fresh orange juice or fresh apple juice. Soak some raisins, too separately. Mix in a blender. Add passion fruit and fresh orange juice. Mix well so it will be creamy. Place in freezer for a 1/2 hour before serving. I've never met a soul yet that did not like this delicious shake. Eat it with a small spoon so you can savor every bite.

My Favorite Gazpacho Soup

Place celery, carrots, cucumbers, radishes, parsley, garlic, onions, red peppers and dill in a blender with lots of fresh, ripe tomatoes. Blend slowly. When it's a soup consistency, pour it into a glass bowl and chill. When ready to serve, add olive or flax seed oil, finely chopped chives, your favorite diced crunchy veggies, and serve. It is very nutritious and great on a hot summer day. Use the veggies you like.

Raw - Essene Bread

Don't turn your nose up yet! This raw bread is sun-baked and delicious. It's probably the most seductive of raw foods. The recipe calls for sprouted grains, easily digested and much more nutritious. You can bake it in the sun, or leave it on your counter for a day at room temperature. The point is not to heat above 100° F so the vital enzymes and vitamins become inactivated. There are many different variations of this recipe and you can make it up as you go!

The main ingredient is organic wheat or millet, soaked overnight, then sprouted for a few days. Grind the sprouts in a food processor. Add a bit of oil and form into a ball. Place it on a breadboard sprinkled with wheat germ to prevent the dough from sticking. Role the dough into very thin sheets with a rolling pin dusted with wheat germ or ground sesame seeds. Press it onto a thin, flat cookie sheet or tray and set it out for six - twelve hours in the sun, flipping it over on both sides. Make sure it's not so big you can't flip it easily with a spatula. You may choose to make it tortilla size in order to handle it easier. You can leave it on your kitchen counter in the house, too.

You can add a sprinkle of herbs, vegetables, or seasoning before blending the dough. This is the only bread you won't feel guilty about eating. When I gave up bread I felt bad thinking how hard it would be living without the staple food of my life. With this raw bread, I don't feel like I'm missing a thing!

You can use millet or any grain to make bread like this that is also good for you. Millet is one of the best grains since it's one of the few that's alkaline, plus, it contains all eight essential amino acids. You can sprout or soak it.

Volumes have been written on the subject of eating but the big secret is to keep it simple and fresh. We don't live to eat, we eat to live. Food that nourishes you doesn't plug you up and make you tired. Less is more. Quality is the key - fresh.

My son Jesse is a raw foodist and was healed totally of various ill health symptoms. I must say that if you have ever had any health problems they will vanish through a fresh-raw diet. That is just the beginning of many wonderful things awaiting you. The most exciting is total, clear thinking, kindness, enlightenment, peace-oneness. If you only try this for thirty days, says Jesse, you will never go back to the old ways.

Slowly things will start to unfold for you. Confidence builds up, you feel different and you can't quite put your finger on it. From this point on you become comfortable that you are doing the right thing, so you don't have the need to convince anyone to do what you are doing and no one can talk you out of it.

Many books with recipes are listed in the back of this book. I also teach a four-day class in making good foods. The location varies.

Check my website: www.thecureisinthecause.org.
www.thecureisinthecause.com

Children and Raw Food

One of my deepest concerns is children and how to introduce them to, and interest them in, eating more raw foods. An interesting point to bring up is that breast-fed babies have a natural desire for wholesome food from birth. Also what kind of food a pregnant mother eats is a major factor that will determine a child's likes and dislikes later in life. It's when their tastes get altered by commercial baby foods loaded with sugar, salt, artificial flavors and preservatives that children loose the instinctive knowledge of which foods they need. Did you even notice how young children will eat the same thing over and over until their body has had enough of whatever nutrient it needs for that stage of development? Start them right from the very beginning on natural raw foods and they will never crave junk food.

However when you try to correct the eating habits of an older child the task is more difficult. Their tastes have been partially formed. All likes and dislikes are learned so they will need to unlearn them. Some foods are extremely addictive and there are children who will learn to like only artificial flavorings and who will literally be allergic to fresh fruits and vegetables due to enzyme depletion and altered taste buds.

It's always worthwhile to point out good fruits and vegetables so children can understand why they are important, and how damaging artificial and junk foods are. Persistence and patience are keys. Be a good example and do not keep any junk food around. Slowly they'll start to enjoy the variety. Just don't make a big deal out of it.

Many parents give their children snacks that are junk. The kids get filled up on them and then don't want to eat their main meal, even if it's food they like and is good for them. Give your children the opportunity to eat right. Have fresh carrots, apples, celery, and an array of raw nut butter dips handy. They can make a meal out of this type of snacking. Cut melons into cubes and serve with a cocktail-type toothpick. Make eating fun. Apple slices with almond butter are just about irresistible to every kid. Variety is important and organic food is the key.

Show children how to grow their own garden so they can see how the plants they eat grow from seeds. Nothing can be as delicious and satisfying as a freshly picked tomato or carrot from his or her own garden, one they've tended, watered and watched grow. They also can enjoy sprouts that they sprouted themselves. When they go to school pack them fresh fruits and veggies, Essene bread, avocados, and some "soaked" nuts and seeds for lunch.

When my youngest son was in second grade he told me all the kids laughed at his avocado sandwich. He wanted to try a school lunch instead, so he did. He became ill from eating cafeteria food and never wanted to try it again. Kids need to experience different things. Give them a chance. Do it gradually and with love.

It is the same thing with restaurant food or family parties. Let children try different things and you will see they will return to good food, especially when it makes them feel good. When invited to a party, always ask if you can bring your favorite salad and hors-d'œuvre. Sometimes that's all you may end up eating. One thing I've noticed is that people usually do not look in your plate so you can hide whatever they "force" on you under your salad. Don't make a big deal out of saying "no" or explaining why you don't want what's being offered. Change the subject unless they're seriously interested in nutrition.

When traveling, carry a few apples and a jar of sprouts completely ready to eat. They can grow while traveling, and can be put in a salad when you get to a restaurant. Some almonds or sunflower or pumpkin seeds and avocados are good to bring and travel well, too. The avocados will ripen on the way to where you're going. Kids love to snack on fruits, nuts and seeds when traveling.

When it comes to kids and good food it is of most importance not to force them to eat what they don't like but rather to make them aware and understand why food has everything to do with their physical, mental and spiritual health. As a parent or teacher, if you provide proper healthy choices and trust in a child's intuition and connection with their higher self, they will instinctively choose the right path. Good raw vibrant food. Make sure that they are available at all times so when kids get hungry, it will be there for them and they will not have a chance to fill up on junk food first. You are responsible for their choices now.

Perfect main dishes for lunch or dinner

Grated carrots topped with sunflower seeds, raisins, dried figs, celery, surrounded by a border of onions mixed with greens on the plate. Put tomatoes or black olives, grated red cabbage or use your imagination!

Try avocado, ripe olives, fresh tomato and chives on Essene herb bread, with a side of mushrooms stuffed with garlic and sprouted alfalfa.

Apple slices and celery dipped in sesame butter, sprinkled with wheat germ or walnuts, or dried figs with dandelion flowers.

Mix the leaves of *young* weeds from your garden with shredded cabbage and shredded carrots. Add lots of garlic, lemon and chopped almonds or filberts (hazelnuts).

Be creative and don't limit yourself to any particular combination.

When you're on a transition diet you need to take time to go more raw. Don't rush it.

You can make wild brown rice in the evening and use it during the next day for breakfast, lunch or dinner. Make the salad of your choice and mix in some rice. Very tasty and stops those junk food cravings cold. Millet can be used in place of rice, too.

You can make excellent raw desserts. Mix dried raisins or dates with almonds, walnuts, sesame seeds, sunflower seeds, fresh orange juice and lemon peel in a food processor and blend it well. Shape it and roll it in shredded organic coconut or carob powder. You'll never want another donut or cookie again.

What is nice about being aware of what you eat is that you will never need a doctor (other than for accidents) or any drugs. You will not need to treat any symptoms - there won't be any.

No hospital bills, prescription refills or insurance to pay. Your best insurance is good organic food.

If you would like to be on our mailing list, please find Dr. Ruza Bogdanovich's address in the back of the book or send an email: drruza@hotmail.com.

Also take a look at David Wolfe's web site for books on raw food and other natural health subjects:
http://www.rawfood.com.

Take it easy

When you change your old ways for the better you have to do it slowly. Start with introducing more and more fresh fruits and vegetables into your diet and choose the ones you like. If you have been on the average American diet, or for that matter any cooked diet you can change by starting with fresh, raw juices without any problems. If you do all raw at once, instead of slowly tapering into it, you might end up with a healing crisis, as I mentioned earlier. Your body will flood a lifetime's accumulations of toxins and wastes into your bloodstream suddenly. That can result in headaches, aches and pains, nausea, tiredness, and irritability. The severity all depends on the state of your health and your body as to how the cleansing reaction will affect you: completely unnoticed, mild or severe. So start slowly.

Constant desire for food and stimulants means an enervated state of the body brought on by over indulgence – over stimulation and burden on all organs. Eating without real hunger; eating when sick or uncomfortable; eating at off hours or between meals; eating until uncomfortable. A driving desire for food three times a day means enervation. Trouble is only around the corner. As they say – the wise will get busy and correct appetite. Less is more.

Fasting is the best, easiest and surest way to cure any disease. By fasting your body, you get rid of mucous build-up and the accumulation of stored toxins.

Be sure to get plenty of rest, fresh air, sun exposure and skin brush every day so you can eliminate the toxins through your skin and help other elimination channels with a heavy burden. Start by eating raw salad every day and drink fresh juice (fruit or vegetable). Drink fresh herbal sun tea instead of coffee. If you drink three cups of coffee every day, trade one for herb tea at first. Slowly switch to two cups and then replace all three. Begin to eliminate foods that are very bad for you: milk, butter, meat, pastries, bread, sugar, junk and fast foods. Little by little you will notice you are feeling more energy. Finally you won't need any more convincing because you will start to become more alive, enthusiastic, happy, creative and brimming with peace and contentment.

If you are filled with anxiety and stress look for the possible cause of it, resolve it, eliminate it. Be sure your diet includes plenty of raw foods rich in B vitamins. Raw wheat germ, rice, lentils, sprouts, parsley, peas and beans and all sorts of fresh fruits and vegetables and most importantly balance your life with physical, mental, spiritual, emotional and nontoxic lifestyle. Remember you are what you eat, breath, think, drink and do.

We get toxic from the outside environment and from the inside environment, from the food we eat, with every meal of the day. If you have a health problem, you must consider any and all of these culprits before you can get better. There are many and we must get to the real root – truth, in order to get free from any degenerative disease or cancer of any kind. What is that something that is causing your problem? You must find out **exactly** what it is or the cure will not be accomplished. **The cure is in the cause.**

One fantastic bonus to eating fresh food is that there aren't any dirty pots and pans to scrub or wash. You will notice you have extra time to read or enjoy your hobbies on top of feeling more energy, mentally and physically. A miracle, you may feel a sense of intuitive insight that you're on the right path.

"What more can be asked of a health system than that it simplifies the cause of disease, making it understandable to open-lay minds. If the reader will read or study in order to understand it he can know what causes disease and knowing the cause, it will be an easy matter to avoid developing disease; but if imprudence brings on disease, he has the knowledge of how to overcome it."

J. H. Tilden, MD

Why start with fresh fruits?

Fruits are the easiest to digest and are loaded with enzymes, oxygen and water. Fruits are a natural laxative, and a wonderful intestinal broom to sweep your canals clear. Fruits are alkaline-forming, while the stored wastes responsible for aches, pains and disease are acidic. When your body is given an opportunity to cleanse, it will throw off these wastes. The alkaline fruits will neutralize the toxins so they won't be harmful, plus expel them quickly. Fruits are also high in potassium content so it will help rid the system of excess water, increase oxygenation in the cells and raise micro-electrical potential. Fruits give us an internal shower.

Grapes

Excellent and effective cleansers for the skin, liver, intestines and kidneys. They discourage formation of mucus in the gut. They are good blood and cell builders. When we were in New Zealand, we had an organic grower bring us 50 kilos (110 pounds) of bunch-grapes. We broke our seven day fast and ate only grapes until they were all gone. I never felt better in my whole life.

Apples

Excellent for detoxification. They contain pectin and galacturonic acid, which help remove impurities from the whole system and prevent protein from putrefying the intestines. Apples have lots of fiber and clean the bowel, strengthen the liver, and stimulate digestive secretions. They're also rich in many vitamins, minerals, and photo-elements.

Pineapples

High in bromine, a very important enzyme that helps activate the hydrochloric acid in your stomach and helps break down protein. Pineapple helps with tissue repair, stimulates hormone production, clears mucus, and soothes inflammation.

Mangoes and Papayas

Both are very rich in enzymes (papain) for good digestion. Papain resembles the enzyme pepsin in the stomach and breaks down excess protein.

Watermelon

A natural diuretic that washes you from the inside. Watermelon lowers high blood pressure, and soothes the intestinal tract and stomach ulcers. The skin of a watermelon (the white part of the rind) contains a high amount of organic sodium.

The key is to eat organic fresh fruits and green leafy vegetables. Use all sorts of fresh herbs, seeds and nuts. Satisfaction guaranteed!

Make old-fashioned candy with dried fruits, seeds and nuts, stuffed dates, prunes, raisins in any combination of your choice. Course-grind the mixture, roll into balls, and dip in coconut, carob or sesame seed powder.

The desire for junk food will vanish as the body becomes more perfectly nourished and cleansed. We are so habit-bound with sugar, meats, and starches that we miss out on the vast array of fresh vegetables, fruits, and herbs. Things will change for the better once we begin to use good food that's mild on our system, easily digested and absorbed. Make sure that you eat plenty of wild berries and any wild fruit.

Green leafy vegetables and herbs that are growing wild and in original organic form are more powerful and are **true** medicine. When I make a salad, I make a point to go outside and pick some weeds around the house and mix them in with the salad. They give you a rush of energy that you will not get with the domestic greens. My father told me that when he was a child during the First World War, all they had to eat was wild weeds, berries and fruits that grew on their own (figs, olives, grapes and carob). People were in hiding during the daylight and could not attend their gardens, so at night they would scavenge what they could. Nobody ever got sick from eating this way. Old people got better even though many were centenarians.

Fermented Vegetables

Fermentation is a natural process of culturing friendly bacteria in food. Friendly bacteria such as acidophilus, bifidus, lactobacillus, koji, miso and all others are very helpful for better digestion and assimilation of food. The friendly bacteria live in the digestive tract and break down the food in tiny particles so it can be absorbed to feed our bodies. Bad bacteria (bacillus) also get in our body. One way to get rid of them is to have plenty of good bacteria so things don't get out of balance. Many cultured products can be easily made such as sauerkraut, kim-chee, seed and nut cheeses, rejuvelac and tofu. Fermented foods are considered living foods, live bacteria flourishes in it and contains organisms that can live in the body of an animal in a symbiotic relationship and are good for you.

Homemade Sauerkraut

Shred red or green cabbage in a food processor. Add real salt (Celtic salt), mix well and put it in a glass jar. If you want to you may also add some water. You may add other vegetables such as green onions, carrots, garlic, bell peppers, etc. Leave it at room temperature for two to three days with a lid lightly covering it. Every day tip the jar up and down a couple of times. After the third day it is ready to eat and if you have leftovers, refrigerate. It keeps for months in the refrigerator. You can add raw sauerkraut to many salads or just eat it plain with a dash of olive oil or flax seed oil.

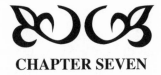

CHAPTER SEVEN

Unconditional Love

"The heart has its reasons, which reason does not know."
Blaise Pascal

If you can recover the ability to love you can do anything in life. You can salvage and overcome bad relationships, improve your health, create harmony in your life and attain unlimited happiness. The sky is no limit.

It's hard to imagine that you can actually love your enemy. Unconditional love is such that no matter what someone did to you in the past you can forgive that person and move on and by actually doing that you become free. Free of ill feelings and hatred eating at you more than it hurt that other person. "Love for your own good."

I know of a woman who lost her son few years ago in pool hall brawl. Her son was shot defending another person and drove himself to the hospital but unfortunately not in time. He had lost too much blood and passed on. He was a very nice young man who never caused any problems. Everyone was surprised at the incident. I did not know how to express myself to the family that would make them feel any better because I never experienced anything like that. I could only imagine the pain must be unbearable.

The young man who shot our neighbor's son was sentenced to life in prison. He apparently didn't remember what he had done due to the influence of a combination of legal and illegal drugs and alcohol. However there was no doubt he was guilty and that was that.

Some time passed. I happened to stop by our neighbor's house to drop off fresh veggies from my garden and thought they might enjoy it. It was a bit easier now to tell them how sorry I was and sympathize with how hard it was for them to have to live through such pain. I briefly mentioned how hard it also must be for the family of the man who did this. My neighbor pleasantly surprised me and said the other family feels even worse. She told me she and the man's family found common ground in their suffering. In an act of unconditional love and forgiveness she dropped all the anger she had against him and became friends with the prisoner. "I had to learn to love the man who killed my son," she said. *Don't judge with your eyes, look at me through my eyes* as Rumi said.

I read a similar story from Napoleon Hill and heard of several more instances but not much on the subject of being able to forgive someone for such a horrible act.

This is the only way. Time heals, and you must give yourself that time, then let go of the pain and suffering or it will literally kill you.

I have seen many people over the years who suffer from different diseases and health problems. When I bring up the subject of their real pain in family or other relationships, they simply stare and refuse to talk about it. But when they finally do open up, with the additional aid of eating and habit changes, all their ill health disappears and brings their life onto the right path.

Chemical reactions in the body are set up by emotional outbursts that directly result in feelings of ill health. If it continues like that for a period of time in a simmering state, the condition of the body will deteriorate.

People die of "grudge-itis." A long-held hatred will cause the body incredible damage, lowering your immune system, which in turn lowers your stamina and the body's ability to renew itself and overcome it. So in fact you undermine yourself physically by ill feelings eating at you. The disease sets in.

People do suffer poor health because of what they eat and what is eating them. Ill will saps your energy. So do anger, hate, jealousy and resentment. Any negative emotions you feel are making you suffer.

What we need to do instead is fill our minds with goodwill, forgiveness, faith and love.

When you feel anger, tell yourself negative emotions aren't worth the irritation they could cause you.

When hurt feelings arise, get the situation straightened out quickly. Go to someone you trust and spill your guts until nothing is left of that hurt within you. Then forget it. Also pray for the person who has hurt your feelings until *you* feel no more hurt. They probably feel just as bad. Sometimes it's easier said than done. Persistence is the key.

I ask people these questions when they come to see me:

One: Do you hold any grudges or hard feelings for any person? For how long has it been going on? Do you feel that everyone is out there to get you or that everyone is helpful? Do you realize that the disease comes from poor nutrition and the state of hate, resentment, guilt and criticism and the inability to forgive yourself and others?

Two: What do you eat on a daily basis? I have them make a report. (What they think good food is along with new lists of proper foods.)

Three: What is your purpose in life? What are your thoughts all day long? Do you love yourself? What do you do to help others?

I have them say with me my favorite version of a prayer by
St. Francis of Assisi:

"Dear Lord, make me an instrument of your peace; where there is hatred, let me sow love; where there is injury, pardon; where there is doubt, faith; where there is despair, hope; where there is darkness, light; where there is sadness, joy.

"Divine Master, grant that I may not so much seek to be consoled as to console; to be understood as to understand; to be loved as to love.

"For it is in giving that we receive. It is in pardoning that we are pardoned. It is in dying to ego that we are born to eternal light."

Thank you, my mentor Flo Collier, for sharing this with me. You are a shining star in my life. This wonderful prayer has literally saved me and many patients by taking time each day to repeat it.

With this information in hand they will think about letting go of grudges, dissolving resentment and changing eating habits to prevent future problems.

We know that stress is the number-one killer and a culprit in the cause of many health problems. If we hold hard feelings, we create stress. If we hate we create stress. If we do not get proper nutrition we create stress. Get positively creative. Replace stress with love. The great thing is you don't have to be around the person you dislike twenty-four hours a day. In the mean time keep sending them love and they will feel it and so will you, the next time you get around them. As Dr. Bernard Jensen says: "I want to love you for my own good."

When you really think about it, it's ego that stands in the way. When you let go of ego the mind becomes holy and neutral. When it is that, love is all there is and there is no space for anything else. You become connected to the energy that is always available in the universe – Nature – God.

Read the book by Gerald Jampolsky and Diane Cirincione: *Love is the Answer.* Also *Your Sacred Self* by Wayne Dyer.

"Understand that love is the highest truth, the highest principle."

J. Donald Walters

Even though you may object that *your* problems are real - and I'm not saying they aren't - your attitude toward them is still mental. If you form a mental attitude that you cannot remove an obstacle, you will not remove it. When your mind, however, becomes convinced you can do something, amazing results will start to happen. You will then realize the power you would never acknowledge. Attitude is a little thing that makes a big difference.

When you believe in unconditional love, anything is possible. You become much lighter, more buoyant as you fill up with love and great things happen to you constantly because you become one with the source of pure love and bliss. The glow can be seen and felt by others around you who are on your side and are eager to help you, they feel your love in them, too.

"Your vision will be come clear only when you can look into your heart. Who looks outside, dreams. Who looks inside, awakes."

Carl Jung

"The more skill you use, the farther you will be from what your deepest love wants."

Rumi

You cannot buy love or make someone love you, so don't try to impress someone with schemes or tricks or playing hard to get. Be who you are naturally and then you will attract love. Nothing else works and even if it did temporarily it would only be for a while until the truth surfaces, then what you wanted will not be there and you would be wondering why. Honesty is the best policy.

Forgiveness

"He who cannot forgive others destroys the bridge over which he himself must pass."

George Herbert

As Dr. Peale taught me, we hardly ever have all the information that would enable us to make an absolutely just judgment. Some things are hidden from us. God sees around the corners we can't. If punishment is necessary, these are the consequences. We cannot be totally unforgiving. Just because you feel sorry for someone doesn't mean you have to excuse what they've done. If a person is sorry, truly sorry, for what they've done they will want to make amends. A first step is not to be judgmental but eager to acquire a capacity to forgive.

Learn to love your enemies and do only good. Forgiveness liberates incredible power in the forgiven and the forgiver. It neutralizes the power of judgment. First forgiveness, then love. Visualize the problem ended, yourself restored, and the pain and alienation eliminated. Fix this vision in your mind and it will work especially with a prayer. Prayer is an important part because often forgiveness is so very difficult we simply cannot do it alone. It requires the grace of God/Nature in our mind to change our feelings before we can begin to accept the change ourselves. As Norman Vincent Peale says, *"When God and love act as solvent, anything can be washed away."*

To forgive someone for what they've done is the most important lesson in life. Hatred, anger, resentment, grudge, and jealousy set up barriers and deprive us of spiritual power. Forgiveness is a needed protection for us.

Dr. Bernard Jensen told his students that he has to forgive everyone, for his own good. So do we.

"The secret of life isn't what happens to you, but what you do with what happens to you."

Norman Vincent Peale

Feelings

"When we accept our own truths, we become our own healers . . . "

Renne Rhae, artist and writer

Feelings are very important and influence just about everything we do. Sometimes knowing facts does not change our feelings. Feelings are as important as facts because of how they affect us. Your mind and your body are one. Think of how feelings create a physical change in you when something exciting is about to happen. You get those classic butterflies in your stomach. Well, worries cause all sorts of physical health problems too.

Your brain receives signals and sends out messages. Feelings always affect your body and your body always affects your feelings. They are one. Feelings influence the way we think about ourselves and about other people. They affect the way we behave. When we understand our true feelings then we can decide what we want to do about them.

Daydreaming takes us away from what is happening around us and lets us wander into our own world. It refreshes us, and helps us understand our feelings. It's good for us. We all need to daydream - it's a form of meditation.

Everyone has feelings and there is not a single kind of feeling that you have that most others also have. People sometimes feel ashamed of some of their feelings and they try to keep them a secret. One thing is for certain, most everyone you know has the same feelings whether we like it or not, including children.

It is normal and natural for people of all ages to feel angry, shy, sad, happy, embarrassed, scared, jealous, sympathetic, brave or cowardly. It is normal and natural to feel curious, to wonder, to feel bored, to lose your temper, to feel guilty afterwards.

At the same time we are all different. Some have more of one kind of feeling than another. Some feelings make them behave one way while the same feelings will make someone else behave the exact opposite. No two people really look exactly alike nor do they feel exactly alike. This is why I'm not fond of statistics. We sometimes try to hide our feelings. Some people are so afraid of anger they hide it deep inside. When we hide feelings our body suffers from ulcers, headaches, cancers, tumors, etc.

We have a tendency to inherit our feelings and behavior from the people we spent a lot of time with - our parents. In some families you are not allowed to show your feelings of anger because "nice people never have such feelings." This is wrong. But if that is what you were brought up with you will bury your true feelings and won't let them surface in your mind. Those feelings have to go someplace. When they do they manifest as something else.

Feelings by themselves are neither good nor bad, just normal. What we do about our feelings is important. Hurting other people never solves any problems and is just plain wrong. Thinking bad thoughts cannot make bad things happen to others, only actions can, but you will not feel good because of them – guilt sets in.

When a child is little they have feelings but no words to express them. Later they learn the words for their feelings, good as well as bad! You also learn how to express them or suppress them depending on the way you are raised.

Sometimes we have a difficult time controlling our feelings. It's good to talk things over. The wonderful thing about humans is that we want so much to be kind, patient, and sensible. We struggle to be better people. In general people are good and strive to be that way.

It's easier to control a feeling if you understand it. Most people discover that if they can talk about how they feel they can begin to control what they do about those feelings. They let the feelings surface.

How often have you felt that what you are about to do is wrong and you do it anyway no matter the consequences? This is a good time to figure out what would have been a better way to get what you wanted or to have reached the goal you did. You have to learn to manage your feelings so that you don't hurt someone else, or get hurt yourself. When we do something bad it is usually because of lack of experience and awareness. Once we learn truly to do only good, then we feel better and strive to do good.

When you were a child and you did something bad, you

learned from experience this was something you wouldn't repeat. As an adult you understand better and are more aware and therefore make less wrong decisions.

Feelings are not just about controlling the good or bad but showing the wonderful, happy ones and letting them flow freely. When we allow our feelings to tell how we think about ourselves, we truly begin to like and know ourselves better. Others, too, for that matter. When we feel pleased there is no pretense. When we listen to our own feelings we are happy. We *must* listen to our own feelings because they teach you all about the kind of person you are, want to, and need to be. You don't need to be ashamed.

Even if you are shy there are millions of shy people who lead wonderful, happy lives. Give in to your feelings and say to yourself: "That's just the way it is." The key is when you do accept *what* you are without worry you'll begin to enjoy *who* you are. We become free.

Even if you are a born worrier, so what? Worriers are often very sensitive people who care very deeply about everyone. They wish so much for good things to happen, that the deep-held wish makes them worry. And there are plenty of things to be concerned about. We need to work hard, correct our mistakes and to make things better for the human race. We do need worriers who care! Do something about that worry; make the most of it. Being your true self is the key. Our feelings help us begin to find out what that self is all about. They are the spice of life. They make us get out and do things. Compassion is a feeling that makes you want to help other people in some way, some how. Do it! Do it directly, that's where it shows the most.

Feelings teach us about things we need to be aware of in order to keep from hurting ourselves. They help us understand life and get along with others who share similar feelings. The more we can understand and like other people, the happier we will be. That's a big part of love, caring how another person feels because you share the same feelings. Walk a mile in my shoes.

Even in our dreams we are working out our feelings. They may make no sense to you but they are always solving our deepest problems. Daydreaming is good for you. It helps work out feelings that may bother you. We get so busy we don't have time to be alone. We get involved in too many activities with other people, or do so much we get out of touch with ourselves and our own feelings. That can make us unhappy deep down inside. Make time to be by yourself. There's nothing wrong with keeping your own company in fact it's a must. That's when you are one with the Divine.

It happens that we can have opposing feelings at the same time. We both love and hate something or someone simultaneously - for a moment. We can have mixed feelings about anyone. The feelings of ambivalence are normal. It's life. No one can ever love another human being every single minute.

A feeling of grief whether over divorce or death is a shock, too much to realize all at once. For a while a person doesn't feel anything, choosing a state of denial. Only when the person instinctively feels strong enough to face the loss can they feel grief. When people let their real feelings come out they begin to get on with their lives again. They have to! Death especially reminds us how precious life is, and how much we want to make our lives matter. When someone we love dies it helps us bear the pain if we think about what that person would like us to do. Doing something in memory of a loved one brings that person closer to us.

Sometimes we wish we were someone else. "The grass is always greener on the other side of the fence." You know how it feels to be you with your burden of problems but you don't know how that other person feels, and what their problems might be. It's tempting to fantasize someone else's seemingly perfect life with you in it, but once you get to know that other person you'll find out that everyone has problems. We can feel better about who we are and what our life is like if we really make the effort to find out how another person feels.

This wish to be someone else starts when we are children. Parents, relatives, teachers, or others hurt a child's feelings by telling them that "So-and-so" is stronger, bigger, better, smarter, kinder, etc. The child thinks people aren't satisfied with who they are and feel like they want to be someone else. In most cases the parent only wants the child to grow up to be the best that they can be. It's not that they disapprove of the child, more that their minds are too much on future potential than on the moment. It's natural for parents to want the best for their children just as it's natural for you to wish you were someone richer, smarter, or prettier.

When we are younger it's very hard to feel we're different from others. We feel so unsure about ourselves and we think that if we could just be like everyone else we see, we would feel stronger and happier.

When we get older we begin to understand that being special can be very interesting, rewarding, and quite wonderful. We start to like the things that make us special and unique. In any case there is no reason to feel guilty about our feelings.

Some things we cannot change. That's just the way it is. We cannot try to hide our feelings. Being who you are is to do the things that make you feel good about yourself regardless of your age or sex. The most important feeling in the world is being at peace with yourself. Say to yourself this is who I want to be and what I want to do. When you've done that you will become kinder and more thoughtful of others. Life will feel wonderful.

When you are happy being yourself you can feel love and empathy for other people. You want everyone to have the same chance too and you have the capacity to understand others better because you know what makes *you* feel good.

Gratitude

"Its the law that says you will find what you look for. If you steadfastly affirm goodness, goodness will be there. If you affirm love, you will find it. And if you affirm thankfulness, blessings will flow."

Norman Vincent Peale

Why is it that we have trouble coping with problems? Perhaps it's because we're not grateful enough.

It's a law of living. If we focus on adversities, we attract more of them. When we are grateful for life and living, our lives will grow brighter.

Dr. Norman Vincent Peale says to be less of a complainer and more grateful for what you have. All our trouble becomes more manageable when we acknowledge past blessings. It seems to activate new blessings. When we find a way to thank someone for what they did for us they want to do more, and at the same time being thankful recharges the soul. When we are grateful we concentrate on what is good. All good comes from the universal source and that's what gives us more strength and more good. When we feel thankful it connects us with spiritual energy. So when you feel that blast of appreciation or sudden vibration of gratitude, turn it into action. Thank that person in some way, call them, write them, email them, give them flowers or a gift. You will feel a rewarding flow of gratitude, an aura of thankfulness that gives energetic power.

"Mentally minimize difficulties; maximize your strengths."

Norman Vincent Peale

Harmony

"I am so absorbed in the wonder of earth and the life upon it that I cannot think of heaven and the angels. I have enough for this life."

Pearl S. Buck

The first harmony is in health. It appears that many diseases remain a mystery with no known cure, and new diseases become prevalent with no known cause. This is how it appears but let's look deeper and see how we got out of harmony.

Established medical practice is failing to understand the root cause of ill health and obviously concentrates on the alleviation of specific symptoms therefore concealing the real problem, which will cause imbalance to manifest itself in other symptoms. So harmony in health is not able to be restored in the body/individual.

Modern medicine is the best in one aspect of human health and that is in the area of trauma repair. People are becoming increasingly disillusioned. So many end up taking several different drugs to control every new symptom.

Disease is the outward manifestation of inner disharmony and deeper imbalances.

If we do our duty to our children and teach them the laws of their being and how to respect them, when they get sick from breaking those laws, ruin their health and call a surgeon who will cut out their mistakes and the effects of their wrong living, then they have not learned to avoid continuing the cause

Every human being has the potential of self-healing. How does a placebo work? From the mind, which is inspired to heal itself, and from what the body stores. **Nature is the catalyst to true balance and harmony**. Not drugs, surgery, or treating the symptoms. Given the right nutrient, the mind/body miraculously corrects the imbalances that exist within every one of us.

The role of different techniques, doctor, or therapist, is therefore that of a catalyst. There is that ability to tap into, encourage and support the inner resources that will cause the whole to unite and restore a true balance and harmony.

All life is energy in motion. This energy, of which each one of us and all matter is constituted, arises from the source and returns to it. It's always striving for harmony.

All life is movement, and all movement flows from positive through neutral to negative and back again cyclically. Energy has three qualities: neutral, positive, and negative. A system of chakras, or pulsing spheres, whose interweaving energy creates the body. The inter-linked principles become two of the energy movements in the body, a subtle energy of being at the physical, emotional, psychological and spiritual level. That's true harmony.

Every side has its opposite. There is not one without the other. For every night there is a day. Happiness is balanced by sadness, cold with warm. We must patiently take things as they come with all the contradictions. They are necessary for the proper functioning of our daily lives.

The more we stay in touch with Nature, the easier it will be for us to deal with life's contradictions and we won't fall deep into unhealthy routine where we need to depend on unnatural crutches that turn out to be disastrous for our body and mind.

Have you ever noticed how some people just feel they belong and are at peace? Nothing can faze them. No matter what happens, they bounce back easily. They seem to be in tune with things around them, and one with their environment.

Balance is the key that opens the door to a healthy outlook on life.

Food is the foundation of life and life is the manifestation of food. This too must be in balance. So does our physical with our spiritual, therefore our mental emotional all in all. Nature is harmony and it strives constantly for perfection.

LIVING FREE
By Nadine Star
(an eighty-five year-old woman)

If I had my life to live over, I'd make more mistakes next time. I would relax, I would limber up, I would be sillier than I have been this trip. I know of very few things I would take seriously, I would laugh more and cry less, I would be crazier. I would worry less about what others thought of me and I would accept myself as I am. I would climb more mountains, swim more rivers and watch more sunsets. I would eat more strawberries and less beans. I would watch less TV and have more picnics. I would have only actual troubles and very few imaginary ones. I would feel only sad, not depressed, I would be concerned, not anxious. I would be annoyed and not angry. I would regret my mistakes but not feel guilty about them.

I would tell more people that I like them. I would touch my friends, I would forgive others for being human and would hold no grudges. I would play with more children and listen to more old people. I would go after what I wanted without believing I needed it and I wouldn't place such a great value on money.

You see, I am one of those people who lives cautiously and sensibly and sanely, hour after hour, day after day.

Oh, I have had my moments, and if I had to do it over again, I'd have more of them. In fact, I'd have nothing else. Just moments, one after another, instead of living so many years ahead of each day.

I have been one of those people who never go anywhere without a thermometer, a hot water bottle, a gargle, a raincoat, and a parachute.

If I had it to do it over again, I would go places and do things and travel lighter than I have. I would plant more seeds and make the world more beautiful. I would express my feeling of love without fear.

If I had my life to live over, I would start bare-footed earlier in the spring and stay that way later in the fall. I would play hooky more.

I wouldn't make such good grades except by accident. I would ride on more merry-go-rounds.

I'd pick more daisies and I would smile, because I would be living free.

Being in the Moment

Being in tune with Nature allows you to follow your instincts more deeply so you live in the spur of the moment. You kind of do things as they come and become more of an observer.

I was feeding my horses and noticed a wasp that flew to the corner of the stall buzzing loudly. She was fighting with a huge spider. Taking my attention to the spot, I noticed that she was stinging the spider. Not knowing whose side to take or if I should interfere, I just observed the whole process. The wasp picked up the spider and barely flew a short distance suddenly dropping it on the dirt floor mixed with hay. She spent several minutes trying to find it, then picked it up again and took off another short distance exhausting herself. This happened many times struggling to get the spider to the spot by the pipe in the ground approximately two feet deep. She took the spider through the pipe and left it there after a while. The whole process took hours. I was amazed at her persistence.

I called my brother Ljubo, a Naturalist, and told him of my experience. He explained the whole thing to me, why and how these particular wasps do that. After paralyzing their prey, they then lay an egg on top of it, providing the new larvae with something to eat until they develop and are able to fend for themselves. Some incredible intelligence-instinct and power to assure future generations. To an observer it looked like hard work and immense respect for all life's creatures. During the whole process of this incident, I was completely immersed into what was unfolding in front of my eyes.

These are the moments that Nadine Star talks about. Moments of meditation without knowing that it is meditation. To allow time to be in the moment is probably the greatest fortune that anyone can have.

Arrogance

"I dreamed death came the other night and Heaven's gate swung
wide.
With kindly grace, an Angel ushered me inside.
And there, to my astonishment, stood folks I'd known on earth -
some I'd judged and labeled as "unfit" or "little worth".
Indignant words rose to my lips but never were set free.
For every face showed stunned surprise . . .
No one expected ME!"

Helen Gilbert

Helen Gilbert said it all.   It's nice to be aware and humble. In a sense, I truly feel that I'm nobody, some fraction of everything. It's not me or my ego that needs to be in charge of my destiny. It's in neutral and being guided by a much greater force that created everything, Nature-God. Any credit would be to my awareness of this awesomeness, intelligence and wisdom that guides me. Humbly at peace, I am filled with love and my simple message is to all: yes, it is yours, too when you become aware and one with it.

True beauty

"Always remember your true beauty comes from within, no matter what methods you use to beautify your body on the outside.

If your heart is filled with envy, hate, jealousy, and ugly unhappy thoughts, it will discolor your aura for all to see.

What you thought yesterday, you will live today. What you think today, you will live tomorrow.

If you want to live a life filled with health, beauty, joy and happiness, then think only of that which is beautiful, and you will be beautiful."

Anonymous

"Everything has its beauty, but not everyone sees it."

Confucius

"Beauty is God's handwriting. Welcome it in every fair face, every fair day, every fair flower."

Charles Kingsley

"Beauty is no quality in things themselves; it exists merely in the mind which contemplates them; and each mind perceives a different beauty."

David Hume

"Cheerfulness and contentment are great beautifiers and are famous preservers of youthful good looks."

Charles Dickens

All-encompassing wisdom of Nature

I love the way Dr. Tilden explains the truth:

"From the time immemorial man has looked for a savior; and when not looking for a savior, he is looking for a cure. He believes in paternalism. He is looking to get something for nothing, not knowing that the highest price we ever pay for anything is to have it given to us for free. Instead of accepting salvation, it is better to deserve it. Instead of buying, begging to stealing a cure, it is better to stop building disease. Disease is of man's own buildings, and one worse thing than the stupidity of buying a cure is to remain so ignorant as to believe in cures without looking to the cause. The false theories of salvation and cures has built man into a mental medicant, being a slave to a profession that has neither worked out its own salvation from disease nor discovered a single cure in all the age long period of man's existence on earth."

How can science place its own knowledge above Nature's laws? Can a scientist construct a living duplicate of a flower or an apple? Better yet can a scientist create a sunflower seed, only the seed that will grow?

What is the natural process that turns a cherry into flesh and bone? The numerous elements in that cherry organize and perform their tasks and conduct the biological functions of the body without flaws. The laws that created that cherry are the same laws that turn that little piece of fruit into flesh and bone.

Nature's balance.

The enzymes that are in raw fruits and vegetables are made of living cells our body automatically knows what to do with. Our body is made of living cells. This is where harmony comes into play. Not in eating dead food and expecting to be healthy. So raw food heals and is **true** medicine.

I highly recommend the book *Nature's First Law: The Raw-Food Diet*, by Arlin, Dini and Wolfe, and David Wolfe's book, *Sunfood Diet Success System*. Plain and simple I consider David

Wolfe to be a passionate, natural genius and a born-again Naturopath. This is one book I have to say is the best down-to-the-point true in every aspect. I agree with what David says. He is living proof. When you want to help someone you love so much you would do anything for them, you don't have to do much, just get them this book. They will forever be grateful, able to save their life and those of their loved ones.

The only way we can be in harmony is to stay with Nature on her promising path. Nothing else will keep us healthy, happy, successful, loving and free as harmony with Nature.

I recently went to church to light a candle as a gesture of respect for a departed friend but couldn't find a candle anywhere. I decided to stay and listen to the Mass being conducted as I had many times before. I was struck deeply by the priest's words: "Nature is faulty, but God is not. We must fear Him or we will be punished."

I believe Nature and God are One. We must obey Nature's laws or we will have consequences in direct proportion to how far we stray away from those natural laws.

How is God - Nature going to help us if we don't help ourselves, if we don't know how. Most people have a diet that is a major contributor to their disease rather than healing or being in harmony with Nature - God. The choice is ours and the consequences are inevitable. The **Cure** is in the **Cause**.

We need true nutritionists to point out what we are doing wrong so we can eliminate surgeries, symptom treating drugs and suffering.

"It is a wholesome and necessary thing for us to turn again to the earth and in the contemplation of her beauties to know the scent of wonder and humility."

Rachel Carson

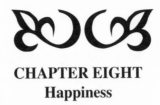

CHAPTER EIGHT
Happiness

"It is not easy to find happiness in ourselves, and it is not possible to find it elsewhere."

Agnes Reppfier

They say happiness is an inside job. When you are healthy inside, you show it on the outside.

True happiness depends upon individual desires but definitely doesn't depend on financial success alone. Our satisfaction is important, not being forced to do things we really don't like to do. Yes, we sometimes must do things we don't like in order to survive but that automatically becomes something that *has* to be.

Very few people do as they desire at all times but to have a job, or career, or profession that is a joy to pursue is a gigantic step in the right direction.

When a person works in a position that provides a joy to oneself and to others, along with a sense of accomplishment, then that person is happy and it will show.

Money does not solve all problems; it's simply part of the larger puzzle. Money doesn't spell happiness, as many people think. Having enough money for your desires is helpful, but if you haven't learned how to live in peace, though there is plenty of money, life can still be filled with constant stress and unhappiness. It helps greatly if the money you have has been earned and earned through honest labor. That means you have provided something, a service, a product, for someone and in exchange have received payment. A moral job that is for the good of humanity and Nature.

In the old days, people used to exchange goods or service for other goods or service, no money involved. The barter system is seeing something of a revival these days. Sometimes this will bring more happiness. I often trade an office visit and consultation for goods like a box of organically grown apples. It brings me joy words cannot explain.

Most people that come to see me, usually as their last resort, are broke from the cost of medication and treatment. I feel uncomfortable having to charge them, so if I know they have a garden or orchard, I prefer payment in produce.

Sometimes people call to make an appointment months ahead due to lack of funds. One woman told me she couldn't afford a consultation until her home sold. She was broke because of a recent surgery and hospital stay. She had lymphatic cancer and was spending her entire income on chemotherapy, radiation and drugs. I encouraged her to come right away, and to worry about selling her home later. She was so shocked I wasn't concerned about payment she actually borrowed the money to pay me!

What makes us happy comes from within. Though we are all one, we're very different in our needs and desires so happiness varies greatly. The variance is because our brains need to be fortified with necessary elements, vitamins, and minerals, in order for that organ to properly function. Money is usually considered the main ingredient for happiness. I believe proper nutrition is! Okay, you need money to buy the food but you don't need to be rich. Like health and love, you cannot place a price tag on happiness.

A very wealthy man came to see me once. He had combination of things wrong with him leading to poor health. When I told him he had to eliminate all his bad habits one at a time in order to get better, he was shocked. Being very rich he could drink the finest, most expensive wines, but the cost of the wine made no difference when it came to healing his damaged liver, pancreas, kidneys and prostate by stopping his alcohol intake and eating out in restaurants.

When we seek happiness outside ourselves it can be disastrous. Bad habits are hard to break, addictions even harder and the more we stray away the harder it gets.

You've heard people say happiness is found in little things. I believe that to be true. Stop and think what makes you happy. Some love to read. Good food makes us happy, too. Some like to grow their own herbs and vegetables, and even more, harvest and enjoy them and share them with friends. Being in the garden close to Nature does something spiritual for me.

There are many things that make us happy, but one thing that applies to all of us is doing good deeds for others. Be loving moment by moment, stay open, no barriers. You are always being allowed to decide for yourself. Be honest with and to yourself and others. How much compassion and forgiveness you have for yourself, give that much to others. Forgive all beings for their debts to you. Live and let live and you will be happy. Happiness is one with love.

Happiness and joy we receive through the act of giving our love and helping someone else on the path of life. Happiness that is based on getting, not giving, is temporary. To give is to receive.

We have to choose peace of mind - internal truth - at any moment regardless of a good or bad experience.

Happiness is the effect of boundless love in our hearts that no one can ever take away. It can never be lost. This is why true happiness is only found by looking inward.

"I don't know what your destiny will be; but one thing I know: the only ones among you who will be really happy are those who will have sought and found how to serve."
Albert Schweitzer

"The great essentials to happiness in this life are something to do, something to love, and something to hope for."
Joseph Addison

Happiness

"Happiness is seeing your work as service.
Happiness is a smile of comfort to the sorrowful.
Happiness is a heart kept open to a stranger.
Happiness is working with other people's realities,
with their natures as they are, not trying to force them
into a mold of your own making.
Happiness is including other people's happiness
in your own.
Happiness is accepting whatever comes,
with an attitude of calm inner freedom."

J. Donald Walters

"Make your life a mission, not an intermission."

Arnold Glasgow

As Dr. Wayne Dyer says: *the present is the only moment that never ends* so we want to enjoy every moment to the fullest. Ask yourself what is it that makes you happy. Do you know what you love?"

Depression

Like anything that needs fixing you need to know first what caused the damage. The cure is in the cause. At times we have what seem to be genuine problems and nothing you do makes them go away. There are bound to be times in our lives when we feel terrible about such things. These feelings are perfectly natural and there is no reason to feel that the world will come to an end, even though it may seem like it at times. Solutions will come in time. We need to do something about the feelings, bring them out and not try to hide them, even under the most difficult of circumstances.

Start by understanding your own feelings. Listen to them, trust them, and you will begin to get to the real cause of your depression. Be in charge of your own destiny. No one will do it for you. No one knows you as well as you know yourself.

One of the biggest causes of depression is a deficiency and disharmony of proper nutrients. The brain needs those in order to function in harmony with the rest of the body.

Depression is lack of self love or a loss of meaning in life. Illness then often functions as an escape from a routine that has become pointless.

Chronic stress syndrome is the mixture of hormones released by the adrenal glands as a part of the fight-or-flight response that suppresses the immune system. When that stress is kept "on" continuously, the hormones lower our resistance to disease, even withering away lymph nodes. Passive emotions such as grief, a feeling of failure and suppression of anger produce an over-secretion of hormones that suppress the immune system so we become depressed.

Our state of mind has an immediate and direct effect on our state of body. We can change the body by dealing with how we feel.

The way we react to stress appears to be more important than the stress itself. Stress can both initiate and prevent illness.

One of the best ways to cure depression is to change your diet to all fresh fruits and vegetables and clear out your system of toxins. Try helping someone else in need. Think how you can be of help to others and forgive yourself your past. Try to be in the present moment.

>*"Disappointment should be cremated, not embalmed."*
>**Henry S. Haskins**

It's very important to understand why you feel the way you do and to acknowledge that you can change your way out of the situation. You are in charge of your state of life.

When you do what you love, you cannot feel depressed. If you are not doing what you love, find out what it is that you do love, and do not let anyone stop you in reaching that goal.

Contact is a very important human need. Get involved with others with whom you have things in common. Some people have no real reasons to be depressed. They are bored with doing nothing.

>*"Never give way to melancholy, resist it steadily, for the habit will encroach."*
>**Sydney Smith**

We can be cured of depression in a short time if we help someone else cheer up. Volunteer. Give.

When you're confused, mixed up about your feelings, you must clear your mind and body of toxic elements and thoughts before you can begin to clarify your wants, needs, or desires. One step at a time.

Sometimes you see people that have every right to be depressed and they aren't. Others seem depressed for little or no reason. They get hooked on anti-depressants and can't break the habit because they don't want to. They genuinely want to feel sorry for themselves. Some lack a reason, a purpose in life.

I've tried to help people in that condition, but it doesn't work unless they want to change and take the initiative. Then you can help if they're ready.

Get in charge of your own destiny if you don't want to be unhappy and depressed. Go to a mental hospital and see what it's really like to not be in charge of your own life. You can begin to take charge by looking within and discovering what is making you feel depressed.

Some people truly believe that their condition is the worst in the world. We all have thought that at times too, but the opposite is true. There are so many people out there burdened by real suffering. You can't imagine how they begin to live through it. But they do. So can you!

Be grateful and watch things change for the better.

Eat good food, enjoy life, do what you love, help others, and be an observer.

"It is difficult to steer a parked car, so get moving."

Henrietta Mears

"What the caterpillar calls the end of the world, the master calls the butterfly."

Richard Bach

"A study of Nature reveals the fact that man must live for service, not giving alms but helping others to help themselves."

Unknown

Death

"There are only two things you 'have to' do in life. You 'have to' die, and you 'have to' live until you die. You made up all the rest."

Unknown

A few years ago I fell off a horse and was knocked unconscious. Our next-door neighbor, a doctor, witnessed what happened. He saw the fall, how my foot was stuck in the stirrup, and the horse dragged me a ways without me resisting. He thought I was beyond help.

I had recently bought this beautiful horse to keep my old horse company, without knowing the new one was a former racehorse. That day my neighbor's niece rode with me borrowing my old Morgan. The last thing I remember was her taking off before I was in the saddle. A racehorse wants to be first and mine took off unexpectedly. I never had control. I can say now the whole incident is wiped from my conscious mind but that day my subconscious took over and kept me alive. I have no memory of any pain. I saw the tunnel of bright, violet light that kept reaching out further and further toward heaven. I was in bliss and peace, truly euphoric and completely content with a smile on my face (I was told).

The rest of my family was away from home at the time but my neighbor tracked them down. The phone rang and before they picked it up, my son told his father: "Something is wrong with Mama. She is hurt. Let's go home." The call was from the doctor asking them to hurry back.

Before it became too comfortable, where I truly did not want to return, I heard my son's voice - shaky and full of fear - calling me. I told him I was fine. It was too beautiful and peaceful where I was, and not to worry, I was in no pain. Then he said: "Mama please, I need you to show me something first. Please come back, don't leave yet." That's all I remember of the entire incident.

I did not feel a thing, no pain at all. I didn't even know what happened until a few days later when my family told me the whole story after I asked why my tailbone was so sore. Everything healed in a few weeks and I forgot all about the incident until this discussion on the subject of death.

Death is something that does not hurt. Before a person becomes unconscious there must be pain, temporarily. If the pain is severe, the unconscious mind takes over and there is no pain felt at all. Before death and before dying pain turns into euphoria and peace sets in.

This is from my own near-death experience and from the experience of others with whom I've spoken. The person who is indirectly involved with a dying loved one is probably in more pain just imagining what suffering goes on. The sorrow of death we are taught, is really not the way it appears to the observer.

Some people suffer much pain and misery before they pass on. It's unfortunate it has to be that way. To me pain is the most horrible thing imaginable. People do not die of pain and suffering. They die a slow death with drugs and surgery. This is where we confuse and fear death. Death is something that does not hurt. Life and death are one - beautiful transitions. In the beginning, we were born out of silence. At the end, we transition into silence. It is the source.

It's how we live while we are alive that counts. Being old doesn't mean we have to be sick and on medication, or in a wheelchair. We can die a peaceful death.

If you do not take any medication your chances of living longer, happier and better are much greater. Once you start to depend on any kind of artificial symptom-treating drug you will never feel better or the same again. That one medication leads to another, and another then surgery after surgery, until you feel like getting older is nothing but suffering.

It truly does not need to be that way. You can actually feel better at an older age than you did when you were younger. You can become younger at any age. Read Dr. N. W. Walker's book, *Become Younger*. The choice is always yours. Go back to Nature and remember that Nature has no rewards or punishments, only consequences.

Nature will never betray you!

"You would know the secret of death. But how shall you find it unless you seek it in the heart of life? The owl whose night-bound eyes are blind unto the day cannot unveil the mystery of light. If you would indeed behold the spirit of death, open your heart wide unto the body of life. For life and death are one, even as river and sea are one."

Kahlil Gibran

"The entire world is made up of only two things: energy and matter. In elementary physics we learn that neither matter nor energy (the only two realities known to man) can be created nor destroyed. Both matter and energy can be transformed, but neither can be destroyed.

"Life is energy, if it is anything. If neither energy nor matter can be destroyed, of course life cannot be destroyed.

"Life, like other forms of energy, may be passed through various processes of transition, or change, but it cannot be destroyed.

"Death is a mere transition."

Napoleon Hill, *Think and Grow Rich*, page 239

Thank god for Napoleon Hill. This truth came to me at the right time and I've shared it many times. Please read *Think and Grow Rich* by Napoleon Hill.

"There is no need to be afraid of death. It is not the end of the physical body that should worry us, rather our concern must be to live while we're alive - to release our inner selves from the spiritual death that comes from living behind a facade designed to conform to external definitions of who and what we are."

Elisabeth Kübler-Ross

"It is not death that man should fear, but he should fear never beginning to live."

Marcus Aurelius, 121 AD

The next piece is an excerpt of a poem from "The Way of Passion: A Celebration of Rumi" translated by Andrew Harvey that has helped many people:

"Everything you see has its roots in the unseen world.
The forms may change, yet the essence remains the same.
Every wonderful sight will vanish, every sweet word will fade.
But do not be disheartened,
The source they come from is eternal, growing,
Branching out, giving new life and new joy.
Why do you weep?
The source is within you,
And this whole world is springing up from it.
The source is full,
And its waters are ever-flowing.
Do not grieve, drink your fill.
Don't think it will ever run dry, this is the endless ocean.

From the moment you came into this world,
A ladder was placed in front of you,
That you might transcend it.
From earth, you became plant,
From plant you became animal,
Afterwards you became a human being,
Endowed with knowledge, intellect and faith.

Behold the body, born of dust, how perfect it has become.
Why should you fear its end?
When were you ever made less by dying?
When you pass beyond this human form,
No doubt you will become an angel and soar through the heavens,

But don't stop there, even heavenly bodies grow old.
Pass again from the heavenly realm and
Plunge, plunge into the vast ocean of consciousness,

Let the drop of water that is you become a hundred mighty seas.
But do not think that the drop alone becomes the ocean. The ocean, too, becomes the drop."

Jalal-ud-Din Rumi

How can I express it more beautifully than my favorite philosopher and poet, Rumi?

Truly when you can transcend the idea that life and death are one and that matter and energy can only be transformed, there is nothing to fear.

The attachments we hold make us feel we will be losing something of a material nature when we die. Today we have so much "stuff" we make our lives more problematic in many ways. Don't be afraid to share some of what you have with those in need and who would probably enjoy it more. Henry David Thoreau once said that anything that he cannot carry on his shoulder with him he does not need. Lighten your own load a bit.

"I look back on my life like a good day's work, it was done and I am satisfied with it."

Anna Mary Robertson "Grandma" Moses

If you are feeling sad that your loved one has departed from you, it's normal. Time really does heal all wounds. But if you feel they may have suffered in dying, I don't believe they did. Before a state of suffering is reached the subconscious mind takes over and replaces it with a sense of bliss that calls you to stay in that state. Whether or not you come back to the real world is up to the power of Nature, if the body is capable of continuing.

"The gods conceal from men the happiness of death, that they may endure life."

Lucan, 39-65 AD

Fear

"Even under the most crushing State machinery, courage rises up again and again, for fear is not a natural state of man."
Aung San Suu Kyi

What are we afraid of, and why? I love the way Kirsnamurty says it.

Fear of authority prevents the understanding of oneself. Under the shelter of an authority, a guide, you may have a temporary sense of security, a sense of well-being, but that is not the understanding of the total process of oneself. Authority in its very nature prevents the full awareness of self and ultimately destroys freedom.

When we begin to understand the significance of self-knowledge is when simplicity and truth come into being. When we begin to understand the importance of self-knowledge, fear disappears. We must make more time for self-reflection, to observe, to investigate and study. Self-knowledge has no end. It is an infinite river, a creative action, and a truth.

"Fear's bite releases a paralyzing venom in its victim and before long, doubt steps in."
Charles Swindale

We must meet fear face-to-face. Fear does not exist on its own. When we face fear, that's when we realize it's only in our thoughts from faulty thinking. Where there is truth, there is light and where there is light, fear cannot exist. Just like a shadow disappears with light, so does fear with truth.

"I believe anyone can conquer fear by doing the things he fears to do, provided he keeps doing them until he gets a record of successful expense behind him."
Eleanor Roosevelt

"Fear: the best way out is through."

Helen Keller

Discover what is it you are afraid of, and bring that fear into the open. Examine the "monster under your bed" in the bright light of day. Once you've taken a closer look at what scares you - and why - it won't be so frightening. Knowledge is power. Fear is the opposite of love.

"Our fears are a treasure house of self-knowledge if we explore them."

Marilyn French

How to purify physically, mentally, emotionally and spiritually

Proper hormonal function and balance in the body system is considered health. Human beings possess higher dimensional homeostatic systems that control all hormones and immune systems **on the cellular level and beyond the physical body** (bones, muscles and nerves). It is not just the physical being but also the multidimensional being of vibrational energy. It interchanges and controls the systems to maintain our health status. Most importantly, upon the intact effect loop involving the hypothalamus, pituitary and thyroid glands; the adrenal, other glands and organs (liver, included) balance the health of each individual cell and their action-reaction without us knowing about it. We must nourish the whole system in order to provide biochemical energy and molecular building blocks. To balance and strengthen the whole system and the health of every cell is imperative in order for the whole body to function in harmony.

Food is the foundation of everything that we are physically. Food also has everything to do with what we are mentally and spiritually, a concept I've been exploring a long time and came up with this fact.

When a person has mental problems, they must have physical and chemical problems in the brain too and in the body also. The brain cannot think clearly, logically, successfully with proper stimulus, if it is plugged up with mucous caused by eating only dead, processed and unnatural foods. I'm not saying all of a sudden we aren't smart any more, but rather we can comprehend something only to a point, but not further, deeper, and clearer. I think this is what Albert Schwitzer meant when asked what was wrong with man today? He replied: "Man simply cannot think." It's almost like we are no longer conscious, something is blocked up and we cannot see simple truths clearly. For instance, genetically engineered food, chemicals, pesticides, growth hormones, prescription drugs, processed foods, etc. have a lot to do with disruption of cell communication. This could all change in time, through eating more organic, raw food, like our species did originally from the beginning. Like the majority of living creatures do. This is the cure for all ills most importantly the brain. Clear mind, proper hormonal balance cause the thinking part of the brain to be in harmony with the hormone producing gland that signal and trigger right responses within the brain and will make the body act accordingly.

We can see modern medicine's dogma has been a failure. There are more degenerative diseases and multiple illnesses now than ever before in human history, and the culprit definitely is what we put in our bodies. We are more "processed" now than ever before. Especially today when a doctor tells his patient that the cause of his disease has nothing to do with his diet. What's worse, the doctor really believes what he says. The doctor cannot think clearly either. Doctors, for the most part, don't pay attention to what they eat. Just look at a hospital cafeteria menu!

When you are internally purified, you can really start to click and remember things. You can see how the mind works and how to logically use that knowledge to achieve health, happiness, harmony, and success. To become liberated from all the past fears, anxieties, despair and finally see and feel the truth. When the mind is free and clear of toxicity (physically and mentally) and supplied with pure organic nutrients, and the truth, we become "born again", thrilled about life. Our purpose and every action that we take seem like the right moves. People around you will tell you that you glow in the dark. The sky is the limit to what you can accomplish and feel.

The connection between health, happiness, love, success and diet are absolutely crucial. It's all one, a fact that you need to know. This is undeniable truth. No doubt about it.

The greatest, yet simplest truths have shaken civilizations to their core, yet to some, the truth appears insignificant. Other observers miss the truth entirely.

Today we are missing so much there is the real danger our own Nature will rebel. Look how our immune systems no longer know who we are. They fight us in their own confusion. The brain is no longer in its proper state of mind, and other major points (organs, glands) it sends signals that are not able to respond with chemical correctness. The cells are confused. DNA, too. Misinformation in communication of the pituitary and hypothalamus - our master.

Maybe this isn't making sense to you.

What is our problem? Our focus and obsessive drive to conquer Nature to make ourselves more comfortable and secure has left the natural system of the planet polluted and on the verge of collapse. How can we go on this way? Now that we have created the means to material security, we feel that something is missing. Can you detect a glimpse of that which is missing? And when you can, you become aware - awake. When you understand your struggle, you immediately begin to transcend that conflict because the energy that you receive is coming from the central source. It is truth - Nature - God. This is the cure for everything especially the meaning of life.

Or maybe you've passed this stage and you know exactly what we are talking about. If so, I hope that you can help someone else see the light.

See the Contacts section in the back and order David Wolfe's books *Nature's First Law* and *Sunfood Diet Success System*. He explains in clear terms how all through mankind's history (all other animals included) humans lived exclusively on a natural, raw diet. Since the rediscovery of fire, humans have destroyed their essential nutrients. This is the origin of all diseases that afflict humans today. Animals, too, are fed processed dead foods and suffer from degenerative diseases like never before.

If we want things to change, we have to change our thinking pattern. In order to do that, we must change our eating habits. Everything that is happening to us is happening with us. We are the reflection on the outside of our inside. It's true!

When we are totally responsible for our actions and ourselves, it forces us to research all the effects all the way back to the cause. When we clearly understand causes, life transforms and we transcend - become enlightened. That's where we want to be. Pure love and joy.

There is nothing wrong, however, with skipping food all together and just drinking distilled water or raw juice for a few days. Dr. Patricia Bragg recommends fasting one day a week and feels wonderful because of it. Through her work she has helped millions of people get on Nature's path. The most important thing is to keep it simple. Read health books.

Fasting is a wonderful way to clean out the extra mucus that accumulates from too much processed food that we ingest. There are many doctors that supervise fasting and have incredible results for most degenerative conditions. Look in the back of the book in the index.

The spiritual part of us is just as important. When your mind is at peace, your body is doing its job physically and your spirit enjoys the way you feel and wants to stay with you as long as it feels right. The brain is the instrument of the soul's activity and obstacles become stepping-stones to a higher way.

A nurse once told me a hospitalized friend would be passing soon. I asked the nurse how she knew the time was near when all the vital signs were fine? The nurse replied she simply knew. She said she didn't need to check vital signs at all. She'd been a nurse for twenty-five years and felt the body was not the same once the spirit wanted to desert it. A body without a spirit has no energy left. The nurse told me it's a magical moment for the patient, and the body cannot be saved, no matter what the vital signs show. As it turns out, she was correct, and my friend passed away soon after my visit.

As you can see, the spirit is happy with us when we are content with ourselves. This is why I feel that the body heals itself. We always try to give credit to some medicine or doctor when in reality the spirit pulls the strings a lot more than we could ever imagine. Life arises from the source and returns to the source. This reminds me of a little prayer I say to help my spirit feel good with me.

"Only for guidance will I pray, that I may be shown the way, and my prayer will always be answered. The guidance I seek may come, or the guidance I seek may not come, but are not both of these an answer?"

This automatically overwhelms me and I no longer need to question or worry about anything. The way will be the truth, and that's always what we need.

When we purify our body, we also need to purify our mind in order to keep the spirit happy.

Healthy lifestyle is what it takes for true healing.

Dr. Bernard Jensen is the light that will always shine for me. In a very simple and wise way he has taught me so much. Just for example, these are a few of the things he's said that have stuck in my mind the most:

"I learned that nothing **just** happens. Happening is just."

"There is no disease without a cause."

On some doctors: "The profession is constipated."

On symptoms: "We treat the treatments."

This is what Dr. Jensen taught me about the healing: 1) Clean out the elimination channels (bowel, kidneys, lungs, skin, lymph system). 2) Flush out the toxic settlements (mucous, debris, fat). 3) Supply the body with proper balanced nutrients (and eat lots of raw foodstuffs).

Dr. Jensen says to start with fifty/fifty and increase slowly until you can eat more raw fruits, vegetables, seeds and nuts. I believe the higher the percentage of raw the better, especially if you're ill. It's not as hard as you think and is so much fun. You will see in the Reference section the names of some good raw-food diet books. Take your time to make the change. Don't rush anything.

If you have any health condition, getting to the cause (what we eat) will help you greatly. This is a true holistic job. The whole body at one time. As Dr. Jensen would say: "When you do wrong, you can't expect right to come out of it, so do the right thing."

Everything has its opposite. Diseases are reversible. If there is a mechanism for it, then there is a mechanism in the reverse direction. There is no disease without a cause.

I like the way Dr. Jensen explains that all toxic material goes to the weak organs and settles there. The bowel is responsible for it, and of the bowel all organs are born. In each bud there is an organ surrounded by the gut tissue.

We suffer the sins of our fathers and mothers for at least

four generations. We cannot continue the inherited diets of our ancestors or we will end up with the same diseases from which they died.

Iridology is the only science that can detect weaknesses. The human eye has hundreds of thousands nerves leading to the brain. The eye is an integral part - an extension - of the brain. This is why it's said that eyes are the windows to your soul. Eyes are the mirrors of your state of internal health. You can help a person best when you tell them the truth about where their weaknesses are, so they can work on strengthening them instead of making them weaker with drugs and surgery. The brain knows everything, and the eyes show everything that goes on in your body.

Why don't we study iridology in schools? We wouldn't be sick so much or have so many doctors any more! Today we need iridology more than ever. It could be one of the best diagnostic tools every doctor, nurse, or health professional could use. Look into it! I teach classes in Iridology and nutrition twice a year.

In the back of the book, you will find the titles of Dr. Jensen's books on Iridology and nutrition. Fascinating science. Dr. Jensen is truly a legend in both fields. He's been doing his life's work for over seventy years now. He's in his mid 90's and going strong, an enlightened being who has influenced me in so many ways.

But, we have to remember that there can be no peace of mind or peace of body without also peace of soul. When you stay on Nature's path and as you realize that, you will fill up with inner energy. Your higher self will guide you and you intuitively know the right steps to take.

Social position is secondary to the spiritual reality of life defined by the establishment. Life is really about passing a spiritual test that you can only discover one step at t a time. You cannot rush it or have anyone teach it to you. You earn it along the way. It's like intuition, you develop a sense of purpose and awareness of your spiritual path - mission and when you bring it into the consciousness, your life will unfold and you feel peace and love and that is all that matters. See how one is all and all is one? Incredibly simple, isn't it?

Prayer and meditation

This portion I devote to one of my favorite philosophers: Deepak Chopra, again from *Infinite Possibilities: Understanding the Quantum Mechanical Human Body;* I like the way he introduces meditation.

"Meditation allows you to dip into that perfection stored in the gap between your thoughts and then bring a little of it back out into your life. When you dive into the gap, you come out dripping with the potential to fulfill all your desires."

He continues, explaining how this occurs:

"Underlying all mental and physical activity is a very deep and profound silence. When you slip into the silence in the gap between your thoughts, you make contact with your real nature and access your true potential. Its the space between every thought you have in your life. Its the storehouse of all your creativity, harmony and bliss.

"The only real difference between meditation and activity is that during meditation things slow down so that your can spend more time in the gap and have greater access to this field of infinite possibilities.

"Like most people you probably spend the majority of your time looking outside yourself for answers to your problems, hoping that someone will give you the answers to life mysteries, when all the time the answers are there inside you. Because your attention is always being distracted outward, you forget the perfection that's already there at the level of your true self."

So take some time out to look inside. You don't have to be fancy about meditation, just do it. Be quiet and listen deep down inside, where true answers lie. Ask your body how it feels. Is it happy? Is it at peace? Is something bothering it? Then truly listen and you will hear a response.

"Deep at the center of your being there is an infinite of love."

Louise Hay

"To pray is to pull ourselves together, to pour our perception, volition, memory, thought, hope, feeling, dreams, all that is moving in us into one tone. Not the words we utter, the service of lips, but the way in which the devotion of heart corresponds to what the words contain."

Abraham Heschel

When we meditate or pray, we allow our deepest yearnings to pour out of us into the universe, to cry out against injustice and to praise the source of love. We become humble. To praise more is to have a stronger soul. Whenever we pour our heart out, we are praying.

"Spirit helps us in our weakness searching our heart with sight too deep for words."

Romans 8:26

Our sighs are the deepest yearnings of our soul and are already our response to the spirit searching our heart.

"I used to sigh a lot before my tears could get wet on my cheeks."

Robert Raines, *A Time To Love*

"Prayer is the song of the heart. It reaches the ear of God even if it is mingled with the cry and tumult of a thousand men."

Kahlil Gibran

When we pray we become humble because we reach that part of our soul which is totally pure and free. When we are free we are kind and give pure love that has no boundary or condition. We become buoyant so obstacles do not exist.

Doing what you love

"Work is much more fun than fun."

Noel Coward

Being aware of what you love and why is the key. Doing what you love is a privilege and pay for that work is a bonus. When work absorbs you, it does not feel like work. It's fun. But it has to be the kind of work that is good for others as well as you.

So many people hate what they do for a living. They feel trapped in their situation, unable to get out. Most people don't stop to think about how their job might be affecting us all.

Dr. Jensen once told me a story about a man who came to see him for health reasons. He had leukemia and hated his job. Dr. Jensen wanted the man to quit his job immediately and told him the job was killing him and his friends too. The man drove a delivery truck for a major soft drink manufacturer. Dr. Jensen told the man if he couldn't quit his job, he wouldn't be able to help him.

"I have three children to feed," said the man. "How can I quit my job?"

Selling soft drinks, that could cause ill health in people, wasn't a good job to have, so contracting leukemia was brought on by the deeply rooted law of cause and effect. Life is a boomerang. What you "throw" out there comes back to you. Directly and indirectly. *"As you sow, so shall you reap."*

The man got rid of his job, learned about the laws of Nature, got on a good diet, and no longer has leukemia.

When we do work we love, deep inside the core of our being, we feel good about it. When we are aware that job is also good for us and for our fellow man, we like it even better. When we produce something of value to someone else, we feel better yet.

Work is the cure for all maladies and miseries, and the best prize life offers is the chance to work at a job worth doing in accordance with love, harmony with Nature and greater good.

Thank goodness that everybody loves something different to do or we would be in trouble!

Always make a point to thank someone for what they do, especially a job you don't know how to do or have no interest in doing. Be grateful for people who serve others and love their work. Show more gratitude when someone does the work they love, regardless what that is, as long as it is good for the earth and her inhabitants.

"Without work all life goes rotten."

Albert Camus

"We are judged on the quality of our results, not on the quality of our excuses."

Steve Fargan

"The sole advantage of power is that you can do more good."

Seneca, 4 BC - 65 AD

What is good for you is good for all mankind. I deeply believe that true goodness comes from the human heart and we are all formed good. The more good we do and the more good we spread, the more it flows. Why would anyone not want to do good? Probably because they are confused and need good nourishment so the brain can respond positively.

"It was only when I lay there on rotting prison straw that I sensed within myself the first stirrings of good. Gradually it was disclosed to me that the line separating good and evil possess, not through states, not between classes, not between political parties either, but right through every human heart and through all human hearts."

Alexander Solzhenitsyn

"Good is itself whatever comes. It grows, and moves, and bravely persuades, beyond all tilt of wrong; stronger than anger, wiser than strategy, enough to subdue cities and men if we believe it with a long courage of truth."

Christopher Fry

"Greatness lies not only in being strong, but in the right use of strength."

Henry Ward Beecher

Being aware of *what* we do is important, as mentioned earlier. We are responsible for what we do, as well as what we do *not* do. We must live with the consequences of either choice.

"To see a world in a grain of sand,
And heaven in a wild flower.
Hold infinity in the palm of your hand,
And eternity in an hour."

Blake

It is man's duty to provide moderately for his family, but anything beyond this may be a detriment to his descendants.

That which can be foreseen can be prevented.

William J Mayo

Your purpose

"Life is an adventure, not a burden. Don't forfeit the only life you have now. Do what you always wanted to do, love it and live it, the way you imagined it. When you glow in the dark you will never be lost, others too will find their way easier."

R. Bogdanovich

We all want to know where we came from, why we're here, and where we're going. A perpetual puzzle! The more we understand life, the more we want to know, and the more we begin to realize we all have a purpose. Unfortunately, many never fulfill their purpose from lack of awareness of body and soul, and sacrifice their whole life for others wants and needs. Our focus gradually becomes a preoccupation with conquering and using the earth's resources to "better our security." We lost ourselves in creating an economic security that replaces the spiritual, and along the way slowly repressed altogether our original true purpose on earth. When we become more aware, we wake up and realize that our purpose is our talent, something we truly love to do, and are usually very good at. We are also sensitive to it - and about it! So we can serve others better.

The sooner we realize our purpose, the easier our life becomes, not only physically and mentally, but spiritually as well. We start to feel like we really belong, we're aware of that which we love, and it loves us back. We glow in the dark!

I used to travel a lot, trying to learn more about life and natural healing. I wanted to learn from the true Naturopaths who walk the walk, and talk the talk. The price was high at times, but I had to do it, I was so immersed in the learning I totally forgot about the world around me . . . including my family and myself.

I was flying from seminar to seminar, taking all manner of classes all over the world. I couldn't learn enough truth. My husband complained I spent too much time "going" and all he did was pick me up or drop me off at the airport. All I did was work. That surprised me. I never once thought about what I was doing in those terms. Sure, at times I did feel guilty about leaving my family, though both my boys were more than old enough by then to take care of themselves. I found myself being accused of placing work before family. I defended myself for a long time. My feelings weren't hurt by what I saw as the complete unfairness of the accusations. Finally I blurted out that my work wasn't more important to me than my family, but it was more important to me than my own life. In that moment, I believe my husband finally understood, because he never again brought the subject up. He must have realized I was willing to pay any price to do what I am here to do.

I love what I do, more than you can imagine. Twenty-four hours a day. It's out of my hands, into my life. I simply cannot change, even if I were to make an effort. I feel this is my purpose, every fiber of my being knows that. It took me a while to admit it to myself, and not feel guilty about it. Now I know what it means to be purposeful and to be one with that purpose.

Few people I know truly love what they do, and I sympathize with them. Dr. Jensen once told me that his wife would come to his office library off the master bedroom at 2:00 am, and beg him to go to sleep. He would answer that he couldn't do what he loved when asleep.

I ask people all the time what it is they love and love to do? Most people don't know, though some like really unusual things. It doesn't matter, if they know why they like it so much.

A woman once told me she genuinely loves to wash dishes. Thank goodness for people like her. I'm very humbled by all the people who love to work, regardless of what they do, as long as it's good for them and humanity.

I met a nice man who was a mortician. He's been doing that all his life and loves the job so much he never wants to retire. I asked him what it was that he loves so much about the job. He explained that he wanted to be the last one to spend time with a deceased person and clear their way to heaven. He also wanted to make them look their best for their families to see when they said good-bye. He told me that at the moment of departure from family left behind he sees in humans a true touch of love he could seldom see elsewhere. I called him a saint. He touched me deeply.

These are not extremes. Do anything you have a true passion for, as long as you feel that you are fulfilling your purpose. The love of work - nothing can compare to it. Quit that job you hate and find the work you truly love. Don't be locked into what someone else thinks you should do. Do what you want - what you love.

Many parents try to make their children go to college and become what the parents want them to be. The parents foster high hopes and later are disappointed when everything doesn't work out, then make the kids feel guilty for spending money on school with little result. Remember, the teacher appears when the student is ready, and many are not ready to do what we expect when we expect it of them. Everyone has to take responsibility for him or herself and choose his or her own path.

Sometimes we try many different things and discover none of them were "it". To get to the point where you can be more sure what "it" is that you want, and why you're here.

Consider this: Try before bedtime to suggest your dreams and loves to your mind, things that make you so happy. That way, when you go to sleep, you might dream about deeply buried desires or certain aspects of a job, work you did in your dream that felt very good, or things that touch you deeply. In the morning when you analyze your dream, you many find a clue appearing more often than others. Ask yourself why, loudly, what is it that you love about that particular thought or thing. Try imagining that you are actually doing that work. You will be surprised that one day, it will hit you right between the eyes and you will never be the same again!

When our two boys were little, I used to tuck them in every night and we would talk about what they love to do. Every chance I had, I would ask them what is it that they love and want more than anything. Again and again. After many years, the answers were always the same. They both know what they love and what their dreams are. Now I am watching that unfold. I couldn't talk them out of doing what they love at any price.

When you do find your true work, it won't feel like a job or a chore, but rather your love, your purpose. I call it a glowing light. You will never be lost again.

The human race goes on pretending that life is about having power over others and exploiting the planet. We cannot endure and survive like this. The more beauty we see, the more we evolve. The more we evolve, the higher we vibrate. Ultimately our increased awareness and perception and vibration will open us up to heaven on earth that is already before us. We just cannot see or feel it yet. Getting to the point of reaching heaven on earth is why we are here. When I was little I felt that, when I was in tune with Nature. Then I lost it because of society's rules, dogmas and theories and it took a lot to get it back, but not until I realized my true purpose and why I am here with Nature. And you can too.

Invitation

by Oriah Mountain Dreamer

. . . I want to know what you ache for, and if you dare to dream of meeting your heart's longing . . .

. . . It doesn't interest me to know where you live or how much money you have. I want to know if you can get up after of night of grief and despair, weary and bruised to the bone and do what needs to be done for the children . . .

Truly that is all of our purpose in life to assure future generations of health, happiness and love.

"I am what I am.
In having Faith in the Beauty and Power within me,
I develop Trust. In Softness, I have Strength.
In Silence, I walk with the Gods.
In Peace, I understand myself and the World.
In Conflict, I walk away. In Detachment, I am Free.
In Respecting all living things, I respect myself.
In Dedication, I honor the Courage within me.
In Eternity, I have Compassion for the Nature of all things.
In Love, I unconditionally accept the Evolution of others.
In Freedom, I have Power.
In my Individuality, I express the God-Force within me.
In Service, I give what I have become. I am what I am.
Eternal, Immortal, Universal, and Infinite.
And so be it."

Stuart Wilde

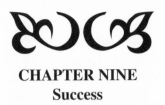

CHAPTER NINE
Success

"Do your work with your whole heart and you will succeed. There is so little competition."
Elbert Hubbard

Remember, for every action there is an equal and opposite reaction. Success and simplicity are one. Once things become too complicated we tend to overlook the main point, become confused and give up.

"Our life is frittered away by detail ... Simplify, simplify."
Henry David Thoreau

Before we can become successful we need to decide what kind of life we want. We must find what we desire by asking ourselves what we wish most, and then live in accordance with the answer we obtain. When we wish, want, desire something to the point we think about it all the time, by imagining it accomplished, and by trying it over and over again, we become good at it. It becomes easy and success is unavoidable.

"Success is all about quiet accumulation of small triumphs."
J. P. Donleavy

Success does not necessarily mean a person is rich but rather refers to the quality of our service to, and relationship with humanity. You know in your heart that what you are providing is causing your success, it's good for you, your neighbor and the planet.

Success follows by realizing that you do not need much. When you feel that, you are richer than the richest person that has not realized that yet, or may never, wanting more and more yet could not possibly use it all. How much truly do we need to be satisfied? We need so little any one person can afford that. Most do not realize it and are suffering from more and more of everything, even sacrificing their health for it. More is not better.

Anyone can become successful. The only thing that separates successful people from unsuccessful people is hard work. When people blame luck for their lack of success, they haven't worked hard enough.

Success is not only about money and power. Real success is about the relationship you have with your family, friends, community, and life in general.

I read once that the first secret of success is self-trust and intuition. Self-trust is knowing something deep inside and then backing it up with hard work. Rise early, work late. Allow yourself to make mistakes but correct them, learn from them. Many are afraid to make the attempt because they fear failure. Many more never try because they fear success. You'll never know what you can accomplish unless you make the effort.

Norman Vincent Peale puts it nicely:

"You must never conclude, even though everything goes wrong, that you cannot succeed. Even at the worst there is a way out, a hidden secret that can turn failure into success and despair into happiness. No situation is so dark that there is not a ray of light."

In order to get to the top rung of the ladder we have to climb one step at a time. It may appear that success happened all of a sudden until you realize you possess abilities you never knew you had. That's success in my opinion. It also has to be our own initiative, exertion and hard work.

"There are many paths to the top of the mountain, but the view is always the same."

Chinese proverb

It's up to you!

"If you think you are a winner you'll win.
If you dare to step out you'll succeed.
Believe in your heart, have a purpose to start.
Aim to help fellow man in his need.
Thoughts of faith must replace every doubt.
Words of courage and you cannot fail.
If you stumble and fall, rise and stand ten feet tall.
You determine the course that you sail."

Anonymous

As with other branches of life itself, success is unavoidable if we obey the wisdom of Nature. It's the outcome of a puzzle put together in harmony, so they all fit as one piece. For every action there's an opposite reaction. We do become what we think about. We are guided by our mind and when it's in harmony with our being you become a winner in all aspects of your life. All in all.

"Don't let life discourage you. Everyone who got where he is had to begin where he was."

Richard Evans

"Spectacular achievements are always proceeded by unspectacular preparations."

Roger Staubach

So many people feel others are successful because of some sort of luck or inherited wealth. I honestly do not believe in such a thing as luck without hard work, persistence, and a constant search for improved or simplified means to achieve something you always wanted. I consider myself very lucky yet I was raised with very little material things. My first brand new pair of shoes, I got as a graduation present. They meant more to me than a new car would mean to someone today.

I learned so much from Earl Nightingale's tapes on success. He compiled stories about a few great successes and what they contributed their "luck" to. Every single one of them credited hard work for their success.

"Success is the progressive realization of a worthy ideal, and the only person who succeeds is the person who is progressively realizing a worthy ideal."

Earl Nightingale

"A man's life is what his thoughts make of it."

Marcus Aurelius

As we are what we eat, we become what we think about all day long. What do you think about a lot?

"If you think in negative terms, you will get negative results. If you think in positive terms, you will get positive results. Believe and succeed."

Napoleon Hill

As you believe, so shall it be done unto you.

We must control our thoughts if we are to control our lives.

We need a goal, a worthy ideal. Deliberately!

For every action, there is a reaction. Nature's Law. We pay the price for not following this wisdom.

We have a choice. As you sow, so shall you reap.

Earl Nightingale says that our mind comes to us free. We place no value to it. Things we get for free we cannot replace. We take them for granted, yet our most priceless possessions are free!

Every one of us is the sum total of our thoughts. You are literally guided by your mind.

The secret of success is not a secret at all. You are what you think so think well about what you want to be!

Grove Peterson said: *"People are basically good. Life is an exciting adventure. We come from someplace and we are going someplace and we should make our time exciting adventure. The*

architect of the universe did not build a stairway leading to nowhere."

As you believe it so shall it be done unto you.

Setting a goal is very important. Keep it simple. Make it specific. Live it. Write it down and look at that goal every day for thirty days. Every day, do something, no matter how small or large, substantial or insignificant it is, toward reaching that goal. The important thing is to do something every day. If after thirty days you haven't reached that goal yet, do thirty more days until you do. Refuse to believe you can be defeated. Visualize yourself having reached that goal successfully. Guaranteed to work. You have to be very specific in what you want. You must become what you think about (want). New habits will follow. Don't think what you fear but what you want. Have purpose and faith. The moment that you decide on your goal, you will achieve it. The answers will come. You planted a seed of corn. You will get corn, not a potato. How unbelievably simple!

"Ask and it shall be given. Seek and you shall find. Knock and it shall be opened."

Act as though it is impossible to fail. Get the book by Dorothy Abram: *Wake Up and Live*.

Don't worry. Hold your goal before you. Be cheerful and reap what you sow. Remind yourself many times daily what you want to accomplish.

Earl Nightingale made it all simple for me. He said we do not make money (only the government does that), we earn money. We provide people with a service or products that are useful. We exchange time for money. Earning money is a result of success in direct proportion to our service. You can earn the money after you are successful. Always place service first, before money, and then money will come. Be of service - create - give.

For every action there is a reaction.

No man can get rich without enriching others. If you want more, you work harder. You gain more, but you always get back what you put out. Call it luck if you like. It's not. It's done deliberately through hard work, persistence and purpose. These are greater laws, Nature's laws that are constant and rigid.

Permanent for you and me and everyone.

Change the image of what you would like to be. Pay the price. Take a thirty day test and repeat if necessary. Remember to act as if it is totally impossible to fail. The floodgates of abundance will open and flow in. You *will* be successful.

Anthony Robbins said people don't know what they want. They don't believe in themselves. You have to find your own passion and be in balance so you can feel fulfilled. Things that move you emotionally, entertain you, tease you, push you one step at a time. You need inspiration, then you can do anything.

Anthony Robbins claims his fame and success is due to coaching others and deeply caring about someone, telling them you believe in them. That's how we are inspired, by inspiring and believing in others. Go for it! Don't let anyone stop you or tell you that you can't be a mentor to someone.

Yes you can!

Once you accomplish what you set out to do, you can do it again and again. You can accomplish new things as well. The sky is the limit. If you have an idea, all you have to do is act on it. For every action there's a reaction.

A very important part of success is to save ten percent of what you earn. Just because you *can* have anything, doesn't mean you *should* spend all of what you earn simply for the sake of spending. Nature is always frugal. She uses only what she needs. There is no waste in Nature. Everything gets recycled and used where it's most needed. Less is more. Just by having more, you can't use it all. Only what you need. Too much of a good thing is *not* good. There has to be balance and harmony in everything.

When it comes to success in health, prevention and diet plays the most important part. As Hippocrates said many centuries ago, ***"Let your food be your medicine and your medicine be your food."*** The cure indeed is in the cause. Profound truth - let Nature be your guide for success in health and the rest will follow automatically.

Liberty

"A guest am I in this world of transient things, unfettered by the entanglements thereof. I am of no country, no boundaries hold me."

J. Krishnamurti

Liberty is the right to choose - to be responsible for decisions made, and to be aware.

All throughout history people have done incredible feats, and thousands upon millions of lives have been lost in search of liberty and truth.

Deep down at the core of the existence humankind always strived to be free and yet it seems as though after one freedom is achieved, it soon becomes overruled by the whims of another party, and another, and another - and not necessarily for the better.

"Let us not look back in anger, nor forward in fear, but around in awareness."

James Thurber

We know what we want and desire, but we are not sure how to achieve it. Perhaps the price seems too high, and we are so tired of opposition that we actually take the path of least resistance and begin to perceive that as reality. This is true in all professions that perpetuate themselves through a system of indoctrinating each new generation, especially the medical profession, past and present. Is what is taught in medical school today the best way, or the only way? This is why medical students do not question the basic paradigms on which their professional future, their everything, rests on.

At one time everyone thought the earth was the center of the solar system and the universe. When Galileo discovered otherwise he was persecuted and forced to recant. This is how it works with a truth that flies in the face of established dogma.

Truth always wins in the end but how long must we wait for it to surface? How many lost lives and suffering continues?

When medicine learned bacteria were the cause of infections it looked for ways to deal with them. Hence antibiotics were introduced, and used to the point where they are now abused. But is it the bacteria or virus causing the health problem, or is it the fertile soil of a weak system where illness begins and ends?

The "war on drugs" doesn't include the real, insidious problems: sugar, prescription medications, artificial flavors or colors, monosodium glutamate (MSG), fluoride, chlorine, tobacco, alcohol and others. Why? Because of the tax revenue the government receives from the companies who manufacture these "legal" drugs. "Who pays the piper calls the tune." We must liberate ourselves.

"The truth takes flesh in forms that cannot express it; and thus its history and ideal always overhangs, like the moon, and rules the tide which rises simultaneously in all the souls of a generation."

Emerson

Each profession has its system of degeneration and is out of control. Each is like a great fraternity: cancer associations, heart associations, lung associations, diabetes associations, etc. Completely brainwashed, not wanting to hear the truth, they live on like parasites, sucking the host until there's nothing left. Perhaps a few strong-minded truth-seekers will survive this onslaught, but the majority of us lack awareness. We are being bombarded with lies on a minute-by-minute basis. We must dig deeper and investigate. Don't let someone else filter the knowledge you need through their own prejudices and agendas.

Nature always wins in the end. The truth will slowly reveal itself to the medical profession. Especially, when dealing with life and death situations. Those who have experienced their own tragedies and discovered, out of desperation, a different way that saved their loved ones will start to question what they taught and turn against it. To survive they will have to wake up because future generations won't have any other choice but to go with those things that will help them survive. Right now the medical profession is in denial. How much longer can this go on?

Drugs are not working, surgery is not solving anything, people are dying of more diseases, chronic and degenerative. Antibiotics, immunizations, prescriptions, etc. are killing us off the face of this planet.

We are woefully ignorant of the truth about how this whole thing got started and got so powerful and so out of control. Now it's loose like a monster, like a cancer cell that goes into metastasis. Like a huge parasite that cannot be stopped before it kills its host. This is where we are today. Wake up! You are not dreaming. This is reality. This is the truth.

How can we be free of medical dogma when in the medical profession it's illegal to be honest? Why is it illegal to have a license to be a natural doctor who cannot possibly harm you, while the medical doctor who is prescribing drugs that will cause all sorts of side effects and possibly kill you from biological reactions, is legal and okay? How can we get liberated and do what's right.

Being free to choose what's best for you and your loved ones is freedom - liberty. To do what's best for you, using your own common sense and Nature-given wisdom. Liberty in all aspects of your own life is Nature's law. Nobody in this world can stop you, has a right to stop you and yet we are constantly being told what to do, what's legal and what's illegal. Things that harm you are legal, and things that help you are illegal. This makes no sense at all and yet it happens all the time and we don't even think twice about it.

We know there's no free lunch but we're led to believe the government will give us something-for-nothing with food stamps, welfare, some college scholarships, etc. The cheese is always free in the mouse trap. Look at the price we pay in higher taxes, not to mention the ongoing brainwashing everywhere from kindergarten to the voting booth, forced vaccinations, licensing requirements and more bureaucratic laws designed to regulate us into whimpering submission.

You can see this with modern medicine. They make the laws to suit themselves and we obey them as sheep. Pharmaceutical companies pay top dollar to fund advertising that fills our heads with lies. Have a cold? Take a pill. Got a yeast infection? Take a pill. Overweight? Take a pill. Heart attack? Take a pill. Loss of memory? Take a pill. No sex? Take a pill. Your child too active? Take a pill and give him one too. And this is legal.

We are in a trap that will be hard to break out of. We are being prevented from having a truly free existence and living the way we want to naturally without changing the world or the people around us. Free to have more rewarding, more special work. Free to stop the government or any organized institution from taking too much of our hard-earned money. Free to have more time to enjoy life. Free to choose what's best for us and our children.

Freedom in any relationship can work only if in the self-interest of each person in that relationship.

I love the way **Harry Browne** puts it in his 1974 best-seller, *How I Found Freedom in an Unfree World:*

"Groups don't think, act, or have motivations, only individuals do. Each individual is different from every other. How can we fit in one world? There isn't much in common when you extend the relationship beyond the one of mutual self-interest, so someone will have to sacrifice. Any relationship should last only if and as long as it is beneficial for each party. Intimacy needs to be cultivated and nourished."

The right to choose and to be responsible for the decision you make is the ultimate freedom in all aspects of our lives.

In health, too! The good news is when you choose alive, raw food, you are choosing life and no disease can win over your healthy body.

In today's world even when you want to do good, it's against some man-made law. How can we expect things to be better without awareness?

When you do finally achieve new levels of awareness and no longer have the desire to change yourself any more for anyone else, that's when you become free. Do as you please as it feels good, as long as you are not hurting or controlling others or Nature.

You are free to live as you want without having to change or wait for the man-made laws to change, or for someone to change the world.

You are for yourself on your own initiative without having to convince others of what you want or forcing, educating, or involving anyone to do what you want. Everyone has his or her own price to pay for doing or not doing what is in harmony with Nature.

It seems as though the only way to do this is to be independent and low-key. As my father said to me once: "Silence is Golden. Do only good. When you do good things quietly, no one will notice you."

Truth can take a long time to surface.

"When man's knowledge is not in order, the more of it that he has, the greater will be his confusion."

Herbert Spencer

We need to be liberated so we may only do good and no longer need to endure the consequences of someone else's mistakes.

If you can only do what you wanted (free to choose), you would want to do only good. When no one is cornering you there is no resistance. When there is no resistance there is peace, contentment and love. When you feel this and allow others to feel that way too, there is cultural transformation, a global awakening. Social position is secondary to the spiritual reality of life as defined by the establishment and life is truly about passing a spiritual test. When you discover the true meaning of life itself you are born again with a totally different outlook on life and you become liberated. You simply glow.

Freedom

"Every great advance in natural knowledge has involved the absolute rejection of authority."

Thomas Huxley

"What right have you to hold on to someone only to curse the dark side of his personality?"

David Viscott

We have always lived in the world that has been forced upon us in one way or the other. From the very beginning we are helpless and had to obey other's rules: parents, grandparents, relatives, neighbors, teachers, church leaders, governments, and the "establishment".

There comes a point in our lives when we get totally fed up. We begin to realize that when we fend for ourselves we no longer need to accommodate ourselves to anyone. Things don't need to be as we once believed. We take charge of our own life and decisions. We have to eliminate all sorts of restrictions in order to make freedom a reality. Many want a free lunch. The only free lunch is in some sort of trap.

Freedom is a discovery of the benefits of acting upon your own ideas and desires and ways to live, as you want to live. According to Nature's wisdom, not man-made laws. Your own freedom is possible and more important than the establishment or society. We cannot, should not live our lives by someone else's code. Only your unique nature is the one that will bring you the freedom, peace and happiness that life has to offer. You have to start living for yourself. Start now so you can satisfy your dreams before it's too late. My father used to say: "Everything in its time." I say the time is now!

Your life belongs to you wholly. You can make it what you want and what you think it should be for you - right here and now without ever having to change the world. That is Nature's Path. That is the wisdom of Nature.

"He who hesitates is bossed."

David Seabury

Given who we are, we can never be one hundred percent free, happy, or knowledgeable, but it doesn't have to be one hundred percent all at once. Life is a beautiful joyous experience as it is, one moment at a time.

There is no all-or-nothing reward off in the distance you must reach to justify your quest. Each new discovery and each new freedom brings its own rewards.

Freedom brings eternal peace and a feeling of not wanting any restrictions upon you, and also of not wanting or needing to put any on others. Let everyone decide what's best for them and learn from their consequences. It's very important to start early so even children can see what the freedom and beauty of life really is.

This reminds me of the psychology professor who totally impressed me in college. I learned much from him about reality and choices. The first day of class, he read each of our names out loud and asked us what grade we wanted at the end of the semester. At the end of the year he asked us to prepare an essay on our perception, our view of life. After reading our essays, he gave us our grades.

The greatest thing about this class was we all put the grade we thought we would deserve at the end, and got exactly what we put down as a final grade, regardless of the quality of our essay. Many students, to my amazement, put down a low grade because they only needed the credit to graduate, or because the class was mandatory for their degrees. I was a foreign student at the time and wanted an A so I could continue with my major in psychology. I worked my butt off on the final essay and probably wouldn't have worked so hard, if I had not given myself an A.

Ultimately, it was my choice and a very valuable lesson. Freedom to act on my own will.

You remember Dorothy in *The Wizard of Oz*? All she wanted to do was return home, but things - and a wicked witch - kept getting in her way. It wasn't until the Good Witch pointed out Dorothy had the power within herself all along that Dorothy was finally able to get what she wanted most. We all have that power.

We are dependent on our mother when we are first born and along the way we learn to depend on others. We feel trapped for a long time and it becomes a habitual way of life. When we no longer need to depend on others we are free, but then others depend on us. We live our life never realizing it's our will that keeps us where we are. We feel that way because we chose, not because we have to. Freedom is knowing the difference, that we are in charge. It's the law of Nature and our right. We feel we want to do, and are free to do, good deeds because good will comes back to us. Good is our Nature when we are in harmony with Nature.

"The ultimate result of shielding men from the effects of folly is to fill the world with fools."
Herbert Spencer

"Many learn slowly, others not at all and still others are put to sleep mentally by truth. I have buckled up against medical superstition of all kinds all my life and I know that clear thinking minds are as scarce as hen's teeth."
John H. Tilden, MD

Being free means knowing the truth. The truth cannot be grasped by all minds until time for thinking has allowed the true idea to soak in. Conventional thinking, fear and superstition have the floor and for many reasons they are unwilling to listen to the other side. When more people demand real truth things will change then, only then we will be free of dogmas and false thinking.

Truth

"Truth never damages a cause that's just."

Gandhi

From *Secrets of Life*, by J. Donald Walters:

Truth is simple

In a sense, each of us is an island. In another sense, however, we are all one. For though islands appear separate, and may even be situated at great distances from one another, they are only extrusions of the same planet Earth.

There are realities we all share, regardless of our nationality, language, or individual taste. As we need food, so do we need emotional nourishment, love, kindness, appreciation and support from others. We need to understand our environment and our relationship to it. We need to fulfill certain inner hunger: the need for happiness, for peace of mind, for wisdom.

Truth is simple.

One reality we all share is our ego, centered in ourselves. Since science will never be able to locate the center of the universe, we are the center. Our ego relates to the vastness around us. We always want to know how our realities fit in with those of those of other people, other egos. We are able to relate to other people's realities more than our own. We become mature and wise, and our vision becomes more encompassing.

Others seek protection from what they perceive as a threat in all that vastness, not only of the universe, but the boundless diversity of human customs, attitudes, desires, ideas, religions, and other social realities.

When we reach out from our egos to a broader reality, our consciousness and self-identity expand. If we try to enclose ourselves protectively against our environment or against other people, our consciousness and self-identity contracts.

The simple fact is that the more expansive our consciousness, the happier we feel, and the more self-fulfilled.

But the more constrictive our outlook, the more unhappy, frustrated, even bitter we become.

The explanation lies in the fact that, although born with egos, all of us are part of, and belong to, a universal reality. We are self-fulfilled to the degree we partake of that reality. And we offend our own deepest nature when we divorce ourselves from that reality.

Truth is simple.

It is ego that likes to complicate matters, so as to feed its pride and own intelligence. Until a person can simplify an idea to the point where others, when they hear it cry "of course", he hasn't fully understood it yet himself.

One of my favorite mentors, Krishnamurti from India puts it nicely:

"Truth is a pathless land. Man cannot come to it through any organization, through any creed, through any dogma, priest or ritual, not through any philosophic knowledge or psychological technique. He has to find it through the mirror of relationship, through the understanding of the contents of his own mind, through observation and not through intellectual analysis or introspective dissection."

In order to know the truth we have to be exposed to it. My father was a news translator. He spoke many languages and his job was to translate the news literally. But that was not what people in power wanted to hear and they would constantly change it. It used to make him feel bad. When he would come home from work we would turn on the radio to listen to the news. My father would say to us that was not what he had translated or what had really happened. He would always tell us the truth and why a politician would want to change it. They seemed to have many reasons for it to benefit themselves but not the public. I grew up analyzing everything because of this and the truth became so obvious to me while others had a hard time seeing it. I was always eager to express it. Sometimes it seemed discouraging that only a few want to know the truth even when it is only for their own benefit. It would be so much easier if we were all taught the truth from the beginning, at home, in school and in public places.

Wisdom

"By three methods may we learn wisdom: First, by reflection, which is noblest; second, by imitation, which is easiest; and third, by experience, which is the bitterest."
Confucius, 550-478 BC

Wisdom is a gift from Nature and Nature's wisdom is all around us. Mother Nature is your best and wisest friend. You probably have not listened to her in the past or you would have discovered her truth and once you do, you will have the most profound respect for her. She is the best nurse you could have. The wise always say that Nature is the way. You have to earn the wisdom with time and experience and because you cannot buy that, you sometimes have no respect for it. We cannot put a value on the things that we get for free, yet the things that we get for free are the most meaningful in our lives, like love, friends, Nature, beauty, etc. It's up to each individual to open their eyes, their hearts, and their minds to that knowledge, then learn to use it wisely.

We learn all our lives, often without being aware we are doing so. We pass our wisdom on to our children and share with the ones we love. The older we get the more experience and knowledge we accumulate, though wisdom doesn't necessarily come with age. It isn't automatic upon reaching a given birthday. We should still take time to listen to our elders. More often than not they have been where we are, done the things we're doing, gone through the trials and tribulations effecting our lives now. Hear what they have to say. Learn from them. Revere them.

Ours is the only culture that takes the very young and the very old and shuts them away from the rest of society, from the rest of the family because they have no "value". How are you going to experience life without them around?

Wisdom knows no age.

Knowledge is information; wisdom is transformation. Knowledge is borrowed; wisdom is your own experience that you earned. Knowledge is ego fulfilled; wisdom happens only when ego is utterly totally dropped.

Intuition naturally gives us right and wise answers.

One Song

What is praised is One, so the praise is one, too.
Many jugs being emptied into a huge basin. –
All religions, all these singing is one song. –
The differences are just illusion and vanity. –
The Sun's light looks a little different on this wall than it does on
that wall,
And a lot different on this other one,
but it's still one light.
We have borrowed these clothes, this time and place personalities
from a light,
and when we praise we are pouring them back in.

Rumi
translated by Coleman Barks

When we realize that Nature is one with that light, we see her wisdom in everything. The earlier you get exposed to her wisdom the easier life will be for you.
A few of my favorite quotes from J. Donald Walters:

"For true love is not desire, the stronger the passion, the greater its demands."

"Peace comes when we love others for their good, not for our own. There is no peace in harboring selfish motives."

"Never complain. Acknowledge that whatever life gives you depends on what you give, first, of yourself."

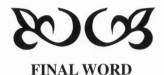

FINAL WORD

Where you go with these ideas will be up to you. You are in charge. Life is an adventure, not a burden. You no longer have to be sick, unhappy, unlucky, etc. given the truth you know now. Don't put your health in someone else's hands and forfeit the only life you have. Make living all that you always wanted it to be.

We spend too much of our lives trying to unravel the mysteries of the universe. We attempt to understand the meaning and purpose of war, poverty, misery and hunger. We end up gaining the upper hand over life through false pretense, lies and dogma and most often don't know or are not aware of it. If others choose to fight political wars with weapons, lost lives and words, it's very unfortunate, but that is their choice. It doesn't have to be yours. Always strive for truth and peace. Truth is simple.

When we truly help others, we help and heal ourselves too. We become overwhelmed with peace, love and gratitude. Nature nurtures and nourishes our body, mind, spirit, the entire being.

Use the life you have to advance awareness and truth (the most important cause that exist) in supporting loving universal Nature - God that created you. Your freedom to choose truth is what matters. You don't need to worry about what others think you should do. When you are one with Nature, she is one with you. If you want to help, help directly instead of through some organized false health organizations and so-called-non-profit parasitic groups that do not want to find real causes so they can continue to survive artificially.

No one can stop you from living as you want to live unless you disregard your own power to control your own life by deciding which information to accept and by making your own decisions. You will always instinctively know when you oblige to the laws of cause and effect. Be involved with people who want you to be what you are and who will give you without sacrifice what you want to have naturally.

You can have a wonderful life for yourself and your loved ones. You too can glow with peace, joy and health. We were not born to die - we were born to live, love, be loved, give and receive.

"Don't wait for the future to change or bring you peace. Live - love and be peaceful in this moment." When you can extend that peacefulness from moment to moment, you can do it from day to day as you live in harmony with Nature.

My true hope is that through the pages of this book, you will find encouragement to want to change your diet and lifestyle toward health, happiness, love and awareness that will set you free.

The cure is in the cause. Any obstacle that you might have can be overcome by looking to the cause. For every action there is a reaction, many in fact. Before you choose drastic measures like chemotherapy, radiation, surgery and prescription drugs, turn to Nature first. Nature provides answers when science fails. Stop harming your body with artificial means.

You are not being punished by anyone or anything. You are experiencing the consequences of your past actions and now you have to change or continue to suffer. You cannot blame anyone or anything any longer.

You may disagree on some points. Let go of the ego that's in your way. The true guide is within you if you allow and admit it. So tell it like it is. You have nothing to lose, perhaps a few pounds, pain and misery. Try what is suggested for four weeks and you will see for yourself what pain-free feels like. I would like to ask you to really stick with it. If for some reason you do not, you will want to start over again. I guarantee you will win when you are persistent.

Your life and your body belong to you, not some corporation or the government. Nature is legal. Most profound changes take a long time. The time has come for us to demand what is right and what is fair, and to protect ourselves and our loved ones from all diseases through true preventative measures. Please join me in getting this word out.

Trying to convince someone to do something that they don't want is fruitless and it will not work unless you want to do it. So I'm definitely leaving it up to you. Just remember that in Nature there are no rewards or punishments, only consequences. Without a clear conception of the cause, disease must remain a mystery - the riddle that it is. You are in charge. One with an innate healing force and inherent ability to return back to balance - Nature/God that created you. She's always inviting you to her silent and innocent beat of the drum.

Over my lifetime a burning desire in my heart, mind and soul demanded answers for truth in everything that ever crossed my path. I found them all within the powerful master/Nature/God and realized that it always was and is within every one of us. We miss it without ever realizing it or allowing it to surface. But when we do allow it in, words could only attempt to express feelings of peace, joy, love and glow. It can only be felt by those who desperately want only truth, and when they find it and are one with it, they are in pure bliss. Nobody could ever take it away again. No man made law or shame, NO-BODY. The puzzle is all in place.

I can't express with heartfelt words how much I appreciate your spending this time with me. This book may add truth that is useful and beneficial to your knowledge and opportunities. You and your innocent loved ones don't need to suffer any longer.

We may never meet in person, know that I'm on your side with Nature. I wish you health, happiness, harmony, love, success, and liberty.

All the best, always,

Ruza Bogdanovich

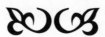

**The author and publisher made all reasonable efforts to
contact all literature sources quoted in the text.**

SUGGESTED READING

How to Get Well, Paavo Airola, ND, Ph.D.
How to Keep Slim with Juice Fasting, Paavo O. Airolo, ND, Ph.D.
Cleanse and Purify Thyself, Richard Anderson, ND and MD
Total Self-Confidence, Robert Anthony, MD
Nature's First Law, Arlin, Dini, and Wolfe
The Healing Herbs, Edward Bach
Healing AIDS Naturally, Lawrence Badgley
Nourishment Home Grown, Dr. A. F. Beddoe
What Your Doctor Didn't Learn In Medical School, Dr. S. Berger
Natural Therapies, Ashley Berke
The Healing Power of Herbs, May Bethel
A Turning Point in Nutritional Science, Ralph Bircher
Key to Yourself, Venice Bloodworth
Many books on health subjects, Paul and Patricia Bragg, ND, PhD
Miracle of Fasting, Paul Bragg, ND, PhD
The Grape Cure, Johanna Brandt
How I Found Freedom in an Unfree World, Harry Browne
Why Government Doesn't Work, Harry Browne
Alternative Medicine, Bunton Goldberg Group
Healing for the Age of Enlightenment, Stanley Burroughs
Living in the Raw, Rose Lee Calabro
The Wisdom of the Body, Dr. Walter Cannon
Man the Unknown, Alexis Carrel
Healing at Your Fingertips, Mildred Carter
Diet and Disease, E. Cheraskin, W. M. Ringsdorf, J. W. Clark
Ageless Body, Timeless Mind, Deepak Chopra
Infinite Possibilities, Deepak Chopra
Milk - The Deadly Poison, Robert Cohen
Anatomy of an Illness, Norman Cousins
How Nature Cures, Dr. Emmet Densmore
How I Healed My Cancer Holistically, Dore Deverell
Your Heart, Your Planet, Harvey Diamond
Fit For Life, Harvey and Marilyn Diamond
Uncooking with Jamey and Kim,
Jamey Dina, ND and Kim Sproul, ND

Raw Diet and Insulin Requirement, J. M. Douglas
Medical Miracle, William Campbell Douglass, MD
You'll See It When You Believe It, Wayne Dyer, Ph.D.
Your Sacred Self, and other books, Dr. Wayne Dyer
I Fought Leukemia and Won, Rex B. Eyre
Immune for Life, Dr. Arnold Fox
Man's Search for Meaning, Victor Frankel
The Great AIDS Hoax, T. C. Fry
Fasting and Eating for Health, Joel Fuhrman, MD
The Health Secrets of a Naturopathic Doctor, Dr. Max Garten
A Cancer Therapy: Results of 50 Cases, Max Gearson
Guide To Enlightenment, Thaddeus Golas
Primal Mothering in a Modern World, Hygeia Halfmoon, PhD
The Healing of Common Health Disorders, Dr. Malcom Hanker
Eat the Weeds, Ben Charles Harris
You Can Heal Your Life, Louise Hay
The Treatment of Cancer with Herbs, John Heinerman
Health and Survival in the 21st Century, Ross Horne
Health Revolution, Ross Horne
Man's Higher Consciousness, Hilton Hotema
You Don't Have to Die, Dr. Harry S. Hovsey
Enzyme Nutrition, Dr. Edward Howell
Pasteur or Beauchamp?, E. Douglas Hume
Love is the Answer, Gerald Jampolsky and Diane Cirincione
Your Health at Risk, Dr. Toni Jeffreys, Ph.D.
Human Degeneracy, Nature and Remedy, Isaac Jennings, MD
Empty Harvest, Dr. Bernard Jensen & Mark Anderson
Iridology Simplified, Dr. Bernard Jensen, ND, PhD
Nutrition Handbook, and other books, Bernard Jensen, ND, PhD
The Science and Practice of Iridology, Bernard Jensen, ND, Ph.D.
What the Eye Reveals, Denny Roy Johnson with J. Eric Ness
Point of Departure, Carl Jung
Super Parents, Super Children, Frances Kendall
Don't Call a Doctor, John Kerr
Nature's Healing Grasses, H. E. Kirschner, MD
The First and Last Freedom, J. Krishnamurti
The Future is Now, J. Krishnamurti

Survival Into the 21st Century: Planetary Healer's Manual,
Viktoras Kulvinskas, MS
Poison by Prescription, John Lauritsen
Vibrations, Owen Lehto
Assault on Medical Freedom, P. Joseph Lisa
Lies My Teacher Told Me, James W. Loewen
Secrets of Mind Power, Harry Lorayne
The Cancer Cure That Worked, Barry Lynes
The Greatest Secret in the World, Og Mandino
Vaccination Condemned, Dr. E. McBean
Natural Therapies, Margo McCarthy
Victory Over Cancer, Leonie McNabb
Confession of a Medical Heretic, Dr. Robert Mendelson
Dissent in Medicine, Dr. Mendelson, et al
Vaccines: Are They Really Safe & Effective, Neil Z. Miller
A Solution to the Cancer Problem, Cornelius Moerman, MD
Invitation, Oriah Mountaindreamer
Murder by Injection, Eustace Mullins
The Power of Your Subconscious Mind, Joseph Murphy Ph.D.
Understanding, Jane Nelsen, Ph.D.
Beyond AIDS, A Journey Into Healing, George Nelton
A New Start For A New Century, Norman Vincent Peale
The Effects of Heat-Processed Foods, F. M. Pottenger, Jr.
Nutrition and Physical Degeneration, Weston Price
Million Dollar Habits, Robert Ringer
Diet for a New America, John Robbins
*Effects of Vitamin C and Flavanoids on Blood Cell Aggregation
and Capillary Resistance*, R. C. Robbins
Bridges to Heaven, Jonathan Robinson
Poisoning Our Children, Nancy Green & Sherry Rogers, MD
The Raw Gourmet, Nomi Shannon
Fasting Can Save Your Life, Herbert M. Shelton, ND
Health for Millions, Dr. Herbert Shelton, ND
Advanced Treatise in Herbology, Dr. Edward Shook
The Essene Gospel of Peace, Edmond Bordeaux Szekely
On Walden's Pond, Henry David Thoreau
*Genetically Engineered foods. Are they Safe? You Decide.
Laura & Robin Ticciati, Ph.D.*

Impaired Health, Cause and Cure, Dr. John Tilden
Toxemia Explained, Dr. John Tilden
Nutrition, Health and Disease, Dr. Gary Todd
Living Each Moment, Ken Treiber
The Nature Doctor, Vogel
Eat Away Illness, Carlson Wade
How to Age-proof Your Body with Antioxidant Foods, C. Wade
How to Stay Out of the Doctor's Office, Dr. Edward Wagner
Maximum Life Span, Roy L. Walford, MD
Become Younger, Dr. Norman W. Walker
Natural Weight Control, Dr. Norman W. Walker
Secrets of Life, J. Donald Walters
Spontaneous Healing, Andrew Weil, MD
The Golden Seven Plus One, Samuel West, ND, Ph.D.
Be Your Own Doctor, Dr. Ann Wigmore
Poisons in You Food, Ruth Winter, MS
Sunfood Diet Success System, David Wolfe, www.rawfood.com
Guide to Healing with Nutrition, Jonathan Wright, MD

IMPORANT CONTACTS

American Natural Hygiene Society, Inc.
(813) 523-3296

Dr. Richard Anderson
PO Box 1439
Mt. Shasta, CA 96067
(800) 688-2444
 or John Cotton at (510) 653-5050 for cleansing.
Web site: www.thefirewithin.com

Dissatisfied Parents Together, Anti-Vaccination
512 West Maple Avenue, Suite 206
Vienna, VA 22180
(800) 909-SHOT (7468)
Web site: www.909shot.com

Live Food Products - Patricia Bragg, ND,PhD
Box 7
Santa Barbara, CA 93102
(800) 446-1990

Celtic Salt (natural sea salt/non-processed)
(800) 867-7258

The Cleanse Cookbook, Christine Dreher
(800) 518-1133

Gerson Institute
P.O. Box 430
Bonita, CA 91908
(888) 443-7766 or (619) 585-7600
www.gerson.org/events

Health and Healing Newsletter
(800) 777-5005

The Herb Shop
(800) 453-1406

Holistic Times
Dr. Clayton
(800) 633-6286

Home Based Education
2269 Massachusetts Avenue
Cambridge, MA 02140

How Healing Becomes a Crime, Kenny Ausubel
American Herbal Science
(800) 633-6286

Hoxsey Therapy (Non-toxic therapy for cancer patients)
Biomedical Center
Tijuana, Baja Mexico
Mexico
011-526-684-9011 or 011-526-684-9744

Dr. Bernard Jensen
24360 Old Wagon Road
Escondido, CA 92027
(760) 749-2727

Grandpa Ed's Organic Echinacea
How to grow and make your own echinacea
Ed & Peg Jensen
(775) 463-4509

David Klein
Living Nutrition
(707) 887-9132
www.livingnutrition.com

Natural Health Magazine
(800) 526-8440

Optimum Health Institute
6970 Central Avenue
Lemon Grove, Ca 91945
(619) 464-3346
www.optimumhealth.org

Prescription for Healthy Living
Dr. James Balch
(888) 447-2939

The Raw Gourmet
P.O. Box 4133
Carlsbad, CA 92018-4133
(888) 316-4611
www.rawgourmet.com

Raw Truth Cafe
3620 East Flamingo Road
Las Vegas, NV 89121
(702) 450-9007

The Raw Life
By Paul Nison
(917) 506-1124 (pager)
www.rawlife.com

Recipes for Life from God's Garden
By Rhonda J. Malkmus
(704) 481-1700

Safe Food News
(800) 7325-3663 (yes, its 7325)
www.safefood.org

Seeds of Change (organic seeds)
P.O. Box 15700
Santa Fe, NM 87506-5700
1(888) 762-4240
www.seedsofchange.com

You Can Heal Your Life
Louise Hay
(800) 654-5126
www.hayhouse.com

The Raw Truth, J. Saffron and Renee Underkoffler
(800) 579-9729

Sensory Awareness Foundation
Charlotte Selver
955 Vernal Avenue
Mill Valley, CA 94941

Dr. Richard Schulze
PO Box 3027
Santa Monica, CA 90408
(800) 437-2362

Systemic Formulas for parasites
(Tell them Dr. Ruza Bogdanovich sent you and
you will get a 50% discount)
(800) 445-4647

Vitamin Research Products
Carson City, NV
(800) 877-2447
Use Code#241085 for a 20% discount

David Wolfe
PO Box 900202
San Diego, CA 92190
www.rawfood.com

For more information on seminars and nutrition classes,
contact Dr. Ruza Bogdanovich
P.O. Box 53, Genoa, Nevada 89411
(775) 783-8735
check out our website: www.thecureisinthecause.org
email: DRRUZA@hotmail.com

Index

To order additional copies of *The Cure is in the Cause – Nature's Wisdom and Life Itself,* please use the order form below:

Quantity Discounts	
Number of Copies	Price Each
1-3 books	$24.95
4-14 books	$19.96
15-45 books	$17.47
46 and over	$14.97

Name _____

Address _____

City _____ State _____ Zip _____

Phone _____ / _____ E-mail _____

Quantity	Item	Price Each	Total
	The Cure is in the Cause – Nature's Wisdom and Life Itself		
	Sub-total		
	Add sales tax where applicable		
	Shipping (see below for rates)		
	Total		

Shipping Charges: $5.00 for all orders under $50.00.
For orders over $50.00, add 10% for shipping and handling.
Outside Continental U.S., call for foreign rates.

Make checks payable to: *The Cure is in the Cause*

Call (775) 783-8735 for phone orders
or Mail to:

The Cure is in the Cause
P.O. Box 53
Genoa, NV 89411
drruza@hotmail.com

The proceeds from this book will help Nature and humankind's future survival through the development of public awareness and truth in our schools and television to understand Nature's wisdom and harmony. The project has already started and you can directly help in many ways by getting involved in this effort to inform the public. Please join me and write for more information.

The Cure is in the Cause Foundation
P.O. Box 53
Genoa, Nevada, USA 89411
(775) 783-8735

You may also visit the websites or send an e-mail:

www.thecureisinthecause.org
www.thecureisinthecause.com
www.spiritsprings.org

drruza@hotmail.com

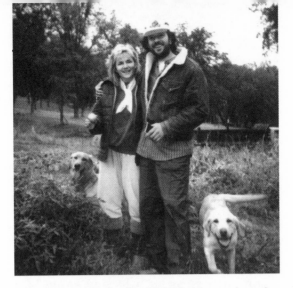

The author and her brother, Ljuba, in his organic garden
with Labs Bulé, and Mac

ABOUT THE AUTHOR

Dr. Ruza V. Bogdanovich was born and raised in Yugoslavia. She came to the US as a foreign student and majored in Psychology and Biology. The serious health problems of her son prompted a career change to Natural Healing and Nutrition. Proud to be a student of Dr. Bernard Jensen, Ruza is a certified Naturopathic Doctor, Nutritionist, Member of the American Naturopathic Medical Association, Lymphologist, Iridologist, and Reflexologist who consults and lectures throughout the US, Europe, and New Zealand. Her articles have appeared in health magazines, and she is the author of several other books: *The Moon Is Following Me*; *Wake Up, You're Not Dreaming* and *Feelings*. She is co-founder of Spirit Springs Foundation, a non-profit organization dedicated exclusively to developing public awareness and understanding of the Natural healing processes. Having been raised close to Nature herself, she has made it her life's work to show people of all ages the truth of cause and effect and how simple it is to stay at optimum health, away from medication and surgery. She is an adamant Naturopath and has assisted many people in showing them that the body does its own healing given the right opportunity and by removing the true cause. Ruza works from her base in Genoa, Nevada.

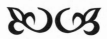

"Everything is gestation and then bringing forth, to let each impression and each germ of a feeling come to completion wholly in itself in the dark, in the expressible, the unconscious beyond the reach of one's own intelligence and await with deep humility and patience, the birth hour of a new clarity .. that alone is living."

R.M. Rilke